Also Available From the American Academy of Pediatrics

ADHD: What Every Parent Needs to Know

Autism Spectrum Disorder: What Every Parent Needs to Know

Building Happier Kids: Stress-busting Tools for Parents

Building Resilience in Children and Teens: Giving Kids Roots and Wings

Congrats—You're Having a Teen! Strengthen Your Family and Raise a Good Person

Caring for Your School-Age Child: Ages 5–12

Digging Into Nature: Outdoor Adventures for Happier and Healthier Kids

Family Fit Plan: A 30-Day Wellness Transformation

High Five Discipline: Positive Parenting for Happy, Healthy, Well-Behaved Kids

Lighthouse Parenting: Raising Your Child With Loving Guidance for a Lifelong Bond

My Child Is Sick! Expert Advice for Managing Common Illnesses and Injuries

My One-of-a-Kind Body: The Ultimate Guide to Caring for Me

Nurturing Boys to Be Better Men: Gender Equality Starts at Home

Quirky Kids: Understanding and Supporting Your Child With Developmental Differences

Raising an Organized Child: 5 Steps to Boost Independence, Ease Frustration, and Promote Confidence

You-ology: A Puberty Guide for Every Body

To find additional AAP books for parents, visit **aap.org/shopaap-for-parents,** amazon.com/americanacademyofpediatrics, or your favorite bookseller or library.

For more pediatrician-approved advice and the latest updates, visit HealthyChildren.org, the official AAP website for parents.

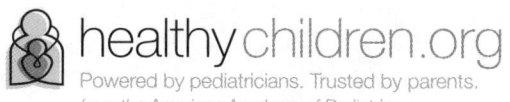

Your Child Is Not Their Weight

Parenting in a Size-Obsessed World

Joey Skelton, MD, MS, FAAP

American Academy of Pediatrics
DEDICATED TO THE HEALTH OF ALL CHILDREN®

American Academy of Pediatrics Publishing Staff
Mark Grimes, *Vice President, Publishing*
Jeff Mahony, *Senior Director, Professional and Consumer Publishing*
Kathryn Sparks, *Senior Editor, Consumer Publishing*
Annika Hawkinson, *Editorial Assistant*
Shannan Martin, *Production Manager, Consumer Publications*
Amanda Helmholz, *Medical Copy Editor*
Soraya Alem, *Manager, Digital Publishing*
Sara Hoerdeman, *Marketing and Acquisitions Manager, Consumer Products*

Published by the American Academy of Pediatrics
345 Park Blvd
Itasca, IL 60143
630/626-6000
www.aap.org

The American Academy of Pediatrics is an organization of 67,000 primary care pediatricians, pediatric medical subspecialists, and pediatric surgical specialists dedicated to the health, safety, and well-being of all infants, children, adolescents, and young adults.

The information contained in this publication should not be used as a substitute for the medical care and advice of your pediatrician. There may be variations in treatment that your pediatrician may recommend based on individual facts and circumstances.

Statements and opinions expressed are those of the authors and not necessarily those of the American Academy of Pediatrics.

Any websites, brand names, products, or manufacturers are mentioned for informational and identification purposes only and do not imply an endorsement by the American Academy of Pediatrics (AAP). The AAP is not responsible for the content of external resources. Information was current at the time of publication.

The publishers have made every effort to trace the copyright holders for borrowed materials. If they have inadvertently overlooked any, they will be pleased to make the necessary arrangements at the first opportunity. Photos on pages vii and viii are used with permission from Adams Lane Photography.

This publication has been developed by the American Academy of Pediatrics. The contributors are expert authorities in the field of pediatrics. No commercial involvement of any kind has been solicited or accepted in the development of the content of this publication. Financial and conflict of interest disclosures for the authors of this book can be found at: https://publications.aap.org/aapbooks/pages/CB0145.

Every effort is made to keep *Your Child is Not Their Weight* consistent with the most recent advice and information available from the American Academy of Pediatrics.

Special discounts are available for bulk purchases of this publication. Email Special Sales at nationalaccounts@aap.org for more information.

© 2026 Joey Skelton, MD, MS, FAAP

All rights reserved. No part of this publication may be reproduced, stored in a retrieval system, used for the purpose of training artificial intelligence technologies or systems, or transmitted in any form or by any means—electronic, mechanical, photocopying, recording, or otherwise—without prior permission from the publisher (locate title at https://publications.aap.org/aapbooks and click on © Get Permissions; you may also fax the permissions editor at 847/434-8780 or email permissions@aap.org).

Printed in the United States of America

9-528   1 2 3 4 5 6 7 8 9 10
CB0145
ISBN: 978-1-61002-854-7
eBook: 978-1-61002-856-1
EPUB: 978-1-61002-855-4

Cover design by Daniel Rembert
Publication design by R. Scott Rattray

Library of Congress Control Number: 2025934506

What People Are Saying About *Your Child Is Not Their Weight*

Dr Joey Skelton offers parents a reassuring, evidence-informed guide to supporting their children's health and well-being amid today's overwhelming and often conflicting messages about body size. Blending scientific insight with practical, real-world experience, this book is a valuable and trustworthy resource for parents navigating these challenges.

            Jamy Ard, MD, FTOS, professor,
         Wake Forest University School of Medicine
           Past President, The Obesity Society

In *Your Child Is Not Their Weight*, Dr Skelton provides practical tips for families while providing calm reassurance to counter the panic and weight stigma that often make managing obesity in childhood so challenging. With his signature good humor and authentic voice, Dr Skelton shows families how they can make positive changes while also enjoying mealtimes, family activities, and the joys of being together.

       Sarah C. Armstrong, MD, FAAP, associate director,
    Institute for Healthy Childhood Weight, American Academy
      of Pediatrics; professor of pediatrics, Duke University

We know so much about the effects of obesity and dieting on the health and well-being of our children; however, many parents and caregivers feel "stuck," not sure about *how* to support the young people in their lives. Like a beacon, this book lights the way for families, guiding them with research evidence and practical, hands-on experience to help them form healthy habits that promote balance.

  Geoff D.C. Ball, PhD, RD, FTOS; professor and associate chair (research),
    Department of Pediatrics, Faculty of Medicine & Dentistry, College of
       Health Sciences, University of Alberta, Edmonton, Canada

Based on his years of experience, Dr Skelton vividly describes the challenges parents feel when trying to make lifestyle changes for their children with high weight. And through stories about families, he demonstrates realistic strategies that are child centered, emotionally healthy, and compassionate for both children and parents. Though the book is aimed at parents, pediatric clinicians should read it; they will find this hard-to-put-down

What People Are Saying About *Your Child Is Not Their Weight*

book full of ideas about how to support parents in creating the healthiest possible home.

>Sarah E. Barlow, MD, MPH, FAAP, professor of pediatrics, University of Texas Southwestern Medical Center; director, Children's Health Integrated Programs in Childhood Obesity; and coauthor, "Clinical Practice Guideline for the Evaluation and Treatment of Children and Adolescents With Obesity," American Academy of Pediatrics, 2023

This book blends compassion with medicine, science, insight, and wisdom. It is so helpful, and so human, and has been needed for so long.

>Kelly D. Brownell, PhD, dean emeritus, Sanford School of Public Policy, Duke University

From the experienced leaders of one of the most well-respected pediatric weight management programs in the United States comes this well-researched, thoughtful, and timely guide to empower parents and caregivers. By presenting foundational supports for family health interspersed with real-life scenarios, the authors provide the practical "hows" so many families are seeking on their journey to improved health.

>Sarah Hampl, MD, FAAP, Kemper Endowed Professor, Children's Mercy Center for Children's Healthy Lifestyles & Nutrition; professor of pediatrics, University of Missouri-Kansas City School of Medicine

In *Your Child Is Not Their Weight,* Dr Joey Skelton and his colleagues offer a compassionate, evidence-based guide that helps families support their children's health without focusing on the scale. This thoughtful and timely book reflects the American Academy of Pediatrics commitment to promoting children's physical and emotional well-being free from stigma or shame.

>Aaron S. Kelly, PhD, professor of pediatrics and codirector of the Center for Pediatric Obesity Medicine, University of Minnesota

This book is a salve for parents trying to raise children who are happy, enjoy eating healthy food and physical activity, and love their bodies. This book addresses weight and food issues of children and teens in a sensitive, caring, and affirming way and provides parents with advice and support for building healthy habits for a lifetime.

>Mary Story, PhD, RD, professor, Family Medicine and Community Health, Pediatrics, and Global Health, and director, Healthy Eating Research, Duke University

Coauthors

Dara Garner-Edwards, MSW, LCSW
Associate Director and Family Counselor
Wake Forest University Health Sciences
Winston-Salem, NC

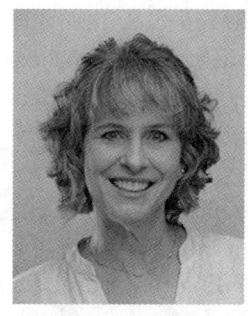

Dara Garner-Edwards, MSW, LCSW, is a founding team member, family counselor, and associate director of the Brenner FIT (Families in Training) program. She received her bachelor's degree from the University of North Carolina at Chapel Hill, completing her Master of Social Work there as well. Her early career was as a social worker for children with HIV and as a supervisor for social workers in pediatric and outpatient hospital settings. She has honed her skills for supporting families with weight concerns through the Brenner FIT program for the past 18 years, including training in motivational interviewing, Mindfulness-Based Eating Awareness, and Mindfulness-Based Stress Reduction. Dara wants to spread the news that all families can get rid of dieting behaviors and eating-related guilt as they find ease with family mealtimes.

Having spent most of her life avoiding pets because of allergies, she is finally able to live with 2 spoiled gray tabbies that aren't causing sneezing fits! Dara and her husband, Chris, have an expanding family of 2 adult children, their partners, and a son in high school, all of whom put a sparkle in Dara's eyes. To add balance to her work and family time, Pilates is what helps Dara with her own wellness.

Coauthors

Melissa Moses, MS, RDN, LDN
Lead Dietitian
Brenner FIT Teaching Kitchen Manager
Wake Forest University Health Sciences
Winston-Salem, NC

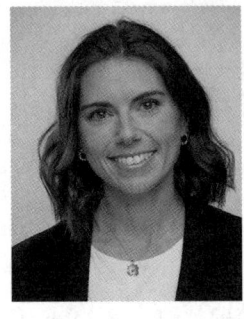

Melissa Moses, MS, RDN, LDN, is a dedicated registered dietitian with more than 13 years of experience helping families navigate nutrition and behavior change through the Brenner FIT (Families in Training) program. She has played a key role in shaping the program's educational efforts and supporting families in clinical settings. As the manager of the Brenner FIT Teaching Kitchen, she leads community outreach and education for students, children, parents, and professionals. Melissa earned her bachelor's degree from Appalachian State University. She completed her master's degree and dietetic internship at North Carolina Central University.

When she's not searching for quick and easy recipes for busy weeknights, Melissa enjoys honing her pottery skills under the guidance of a local artist. A married mother of two, she loves spending time outdoors and believes that the smell and taste of familiar foods can bring back the best memories. Above all, Melissa wants families to know that she's a dietitian, not the food police—and favorite foods are always welcome at the table.

Dedication

To all the parents who grew up dieting and want to raise their children to love their bodies, enjoy food without guilt, and make memories around the dinner table

Contents

Acknowledgments xiii

Introduction 1

CHAPTER 1 Understanding Your Child's Weight 9

CHAPTER 2 Parenting Through Structure and Love 31

CHAPTER 3 (Not) Talking With Your Kids About Their Weight 53

CHAPTER 4 Talking With Children About *Your* Health Changes 75

CHAPTER 5 Family Connection Is Your Greatest Strength 89

CHAPTER 6 Small Shifts, Big Impact: Transforming How Your Family Eats 103

CHAPTER 7 Parenting Through Exercise and Physical Activity 135

CHAPTER 8 Picky Eating and Other Nutritional Challenges 159

CHAPTER 9 You've Got This! 189

Appendix 201

Index 213

Acknowledgments

We are thankful for the leadership of the American Academy of Pediatrics (AAP) for supporting this book and for being a tireless advocate for children and families. We also appreciate all the children and families whom we have worked with over the years and who have trusted us to provide care and guidance as they navigate this difficult and complicated topic.

Brenner Children's Hospital and the Wake Forest University School of Medicine have been a wonderful place for us to develop the Brenner FIT (Families in Training) program, in an amazing community in the Piedmont region of North Carolina. The hospital, medical school, and community have been supportive of a program wanting to improve the well-being of children and families for the long run, not just for short-term changes in weight. We want to recognize the extended Brenner Family (Barry and Lynn Eisenberg, Arthur and Suzy Kurtz, and Paul and Jennifer Grosswald), the Mebane Foundation (Marianne Mebane and Larry Colbourne), the YMCA of Northwest North Carolina, and the Northwest Area Health Education Center (especially Dr Michael Lischke). They have recognized the complexity of child health and have been willing to let us innovate and to let us engage a wide variety of professionals and individuals to develop the best and safest approach to helping families live healthier lives.

This book would not have been possible without our amazingly committed Brenner FIT team, which works tirelessly to support families, trying to find the best way to put research and evidence into practice. They aim to do it safely and compassionately, following our unofficial motto to "provide care that is safe, effective, and kind." A different version of this book was begun years ago by Brenner FIT and led by our expert teammate, Christine Jordan, EdS, LMFT, giving us all the confidence it could be done. A tremendous thanks and appreciation to all the team members, past and present, who have contributed to the approaches described in this book: Lorri Busby, Gail Cohen, Kim Crews, Melissa

Acknowledgments

Dellinger, Sara Ebbers, Casey Foster, Sherry Frino, Sara Glenn, Destiny Godfrey, Joanne Gonwa, Angelica Guzman, Holly Hallman, Lourdes Herrera, Megan Bennett Irby, Christine Jordan, Stacy Kolbash, Jewel Lewis, Katie Maxey, Janet Olivares, Nancy Ortiz, Raquel Pagnozzi, Deborah Pratt, DeOnna Reliford, Sarah Schaller, Ligia Vasquez-Huot, and Anjelica Yancey. We also want to thank their family members, who have supported their working nights, weekends, and other hectic activities to grow Brenner FIT into what it is today.

We want to recognize Leann Birch, Ellyn Satter, and many other clinicians and researchers for their groundbreaking work in childhood eating behaviors and feeding dynamics. Satter's emphasis on family habits and trust instead of scales and portions, and Birch's research on parental and environmental impacts on eating, have profoundly shaped our team's clinical approach and laid the foundation for our teachings over the years.

* * *

I am thankful for my professional colleagues (especially the Sarahs!), friends, mentors, and supporters, as well as all the great people at the AAP. I greatly appreciate Sara Hoerdeman for first pitching this idea to me and encouraging me through the process—you are the best "manager and agent" I could ask for. And thank you to Kathryn Sparks for her patience and persistence in editing this book, which would have otherwise just been a long blog and an even worse podcast. Cheryl Buehler, PhD, was extremely generous with her time and teaching, introducing me to the world of family science. Keeley Pratt, PhD, has been a wonderful collaborator and friend in furthering the study of families as it relates to weight and health, and I appreciate her reviewing chapters of this book. I want to also thank Nisa Taylor for assistance in background research.

Along with the AAP, no one cares for the health of children more than a children's hospital. I was greatly supported by the hospital that "raised" me, Children's Hospital of Wisconsin, and the amazing people who grew our program there, especially my mentor, Colin Rudolph, MD, PhD, who taught me that good writing is not something you are born with but something you must learn. Brenner Children's Hospital and the Wake Forest University School of Medicine have been incredibly supportive of me and our team for almost 20 years, particularly the numerous mentors and colleagues in the departments of Pediatrics, Social Sciences and Health Policy, and Epidemiology and Prevention.

This book is the collective wisdom of a fantastic team of professionals in Brenner FIT. I especially want to thank my coauthors, Dara Garner-Edwards and Melissa Moses; I never would have agreed to do this if it wasn't for their knowledge, wisdom, and endless support.

As it takes a village to raise a child, it took a village to keep me out of trouble. I have a wonderful network of close friends and colleagues near and far who are tireless supporters of me and my family: Raja Chatterjee, Aimee Wilkin, and Alice Chatterjee; Tim Houle; Ellen Vick; Kathy Frontier; Mary Beth and Bob Feuling; Bob Dignan; John and Marsha Grindstaff; and Jana Skelton.

I am indebted to my extended family members, who have cheered us on from afar. I would especially like to honor the memories of my father, Arnold Skelton; his brother Tom Skelton; and my father-in-law, Wayne Patterson—all straight-off-the-farm, first-generation college students who taught me the importance of education, hard work, and family. Finally and most importantly, my incredible wife of 30 years, Dr Kristen Skelton, and my 2 dear sons, Troy and Dylan, who have unfortunately served as characters in the many stories I have told in clinic over the years and who have tolerated long days and nights of this chosen career. I love you.

Joey Skelton, MD, MS, FAAP

Growing up in a village of many caring people and strong female role models, my thanks go to those who have shaped the way I view bodies and food and the work I do as a social worker. One of those role models was my late friend and colleague, Barbara, who taught me what quiet strength looks like—asking for a seat belt extender on a plane with confidence and grace, long before I even knew these accommodations existed. Strong advocates peppered my early career experiences. I found my voice with guidance from my supervisors: the late Chris Weedy, who always spoke up to injustice, and Countess Hughes, as she insisted on the highest expectations for our team. I learned to expect the best from everyone, thanks to my favorite School of Social Work professor and mentor, the late Dr Janice Schopler, who was a key link in my love of social work, keen to welcome my young self into her classroom and field of work. Having lived long enough to lose many of my early influences, I cherish their impact even more.

Acknowledgments

I deeply appreciate the honor of contributing to the writing of this book. It is a joy to write about structure, love, and family meals, as each of these are concepts I hold dear. Family dinners were never a question in my childhood, thanks to my beloved parents, Dr Sammie and Mr Darrell Garner. My favorite mealtime memories were at my grandmother's house, where Evelyn Garner-Ingold's menu always included macaroni and cheese, home-canned green beans, and dessert. Her love of family was all over this menu, and I treasure the memories of gathering around Great Momma's kitchen table.

My humble thanks to Dr Joey Skelton for trusting me back in 2007 to fill a position not intended for a social worker so we could be on this Brenner FIT journey together, and to our coauthor, Melissa Moses, who can literally accomplish anything and do it with excellence, efficiency, and care.

And for the dearest ones in my life who lovingly put up with me day-to-day: my love since I was 15 years old, Chris Edwards, and our amazing children, Nick, Jarica, and Blake. Your patience with this work was generous, and you have my whole heart. Ironically, I owe you a few more family meals that we missed during the writing of this book.

To all the families that have allowed this social worker into a piece of your lives over the past 30 years, I am honored to have walked with you as we learned and grew and got better and better. Cheers to more gatherings at the table!

Dara Garner-Edwards, MSW, LCSW

My roots in a small town, raised by 2 hardworking parents in the tobacco and farming industry, laid the foundation for who I am today. My parents taught me perseverance, dedication, and the value of nourishing the body. Their early emphasis on balanced nutrition sparked a curiosity that would later guide my academic and professional journey.

Studying nutrition in college deepened my love for the science, but it was my second job as a dietitian at Brenner FIT that truly transformed my perspective. I'm deeply grateful to Dara and Joey for taking a chance on me in 2013. Through their mentorship, the support of my teammates at Brenner FIT, and the program's unique approach, I learned to rethink food—not just for others but for me and my family.

Acknowledgments

This work helped me become a more relaxed, competent eater and a more compassionate provider. It changed how I feed my children and how I connect with the families I support.

To my parents, mentors, and colleagues and to the families that've shared their stories—thank you. Your influence is woven throughout this book. And to my loving husband, Adam Moses—thank you for always supporting me in everything I do. You are truly wonderful, and I couldn't have done this without you.

To my children, Addison and Levi—thank you for being my greatest teachers. You remind me every day of the joy, curiosity, and trust that food can bring. This book is for you.

Melissa Moses, MS, RDN, LDN

Introduction

Parenting reminds me of old commercials for the Peace Corps: it's the "toughest job you'll ever love." Being a pediatrician who works with parents and children, and having 2 children of my own, I attest that this is a spot-on description of the job of a parent. There is no one, single best way to parent a child; children aren't born with an owners' manual; what works for one child may not work for another; what works one day may not work the next; parenting changes from decade to decade as our culture and world change and our children get older…and so on. It's tough, and we do it because we love our children—in the deepest way possible and in ways that cannot be described—and because we always want the best for them. So when it comes to raising children to be healthy in a world that doesn't make it very easy, how do we do that?

What Is the Purpose of This Book?

Your Child Is Not Their Weight is a resource and guide for parents who have concerns about their child's weight, specifically if they worry their child is gaining too much weight, they feel their child is bigger or heavier than other children, or they have been told by medical professionals that their child weighs too much. This book focuses on the tough task of parenting children about their weight and health habits, specifically eating and activity, and the myriad of factors that go into each. This book aims to cut through the noise, the controversies, and the misinformation to provide parents guidance on raising children to be healthy and happy when the world around us makes that very difficult. It's written by a team of 3 people, author Joey Skelton, MD, MS, FAAP, and his coauthors Dara Garner-Edwards, MSW, LCSW, and Melissa Moses, MS, RDN, LDN. We focused on the voice of the book from Joey Skelton, and anytime *we* is used, it references all 3 writers. When we say *healthy*, we mean we hope they have eating and activity habits that help them grow to reach their full potential and that could prevent chronic disease. When we say *happy*, we mean we hope they don't feel bad about their bodies, aren't shamed for enjoying a tasty snack, and experience positive interactions with their family and others about eating and exercise. We hope this book will help parents navigate some of the challenges that arise and can make the task of parenting difficult: concerns about weight, body image, self-esteem, and disordered eating.

For nearly 20 years, we have seen how hard it is firsthand, the personal struggle families can go through in trying to lose weight or to change or build healthy habits. Plenty has been written about the health problems of obesity. Very little has been written on how tough it is for families that are worried about weight or just trying to make a change in their eating or exercise habits, specifically the emotional toll, the difficulty, and the stress parents and children experience as a result, which seems to worsen when they try to make changes. We recognize change is difficult, including how it can cause conflict in families and, in particular, how much stress it can cause for everyone.

For parents, sometimes it's pushback from their children or even other adults in the house; other times it's feelings of failure when they try to change a simple habit such as drinking less soda but find themselves still buying it at the store. Making changes together as a family, trying to live a healthier life, should bring families closer. Unfortunately, we continue to see parents stressed, feeling like they have failed, and dreading going back to their pediatrician because they know their child gained more weight. It doesn't have to be that way.

Throughout this book, when we refer to *parents* or *caregivers*, it's a reference to all the adults parenting or raising children in their family.

Whom Is This Book For?

This book is for every parent, grandparent, caregiver, stepparent, foster parent, aunt/uncle, adult sibling, adoptive parent, child care provider, teacher, medical professional, and person who provides care or guidance to children or is part of a family, no matter how you define that family. Specifically, it is for the following people:

- **For caregivers with concerns about their child's weight, in particular if the child is in a bigger body, they are gaining weight too fast, or the family has been told by a health care professional that the child weighs too much for their height and age.** About a third of children fall into this category, and it can put parents in a tough position: they want (and have been told) they need to help their child grow into a healthier weight, but they don't want to cause harm to their child's self-esteem or create an eating disorder.
- **For caregivers worried about the health consequences of their child's weight.** Your family may have experienced firsthand health problems that can be associated with extra weight, such as diabetes, heart disease, and arthritis. It's natural for parents to want to address excess weight that can cause health problems, but the challenge is how to do it without making things miserable for their children or causing conflict in the family.
- **For caregivers who want to raise balanced eaters.** Notice we didn't say *healthy* eaters, because healthy can have different meanings to people. We all want to eat healthy, and we want our children to eat healthy, but there is always going to be debate about what is healthy. If you have a child with picky eating, we will provide some tools for you.
- **For caregivers concerned about the diet-obsessed, anti-fat culture we live in.** With concerns about obesity and rises in cardiometabolic diseases, there has been a simultaneous rise in the fitness industry, fad diets, and misinformation related to health, sometimes by people who are well-meaning and other times by people looking to profit. An extremely unfortunate side effect of this has been anti-fatness, weight stigma and bias,

and the general idea that people in larger or heavier bodies are unhealthy and must have unhealthy habits and that people in smaller or thinner bodies are healthy and must have habits and routines that result in that body. That is simply not true. Children come in all different shapes and sizes, and many factors influence that.

- **For families trying to navigate our world of fast food, electronic games, and social media.** There is a lot of pressure on parents about this. Messages about fast food, gaming, and social media are everywhere, mostly saying they are bad. Finding your way through the facts and judgments is complicated.
- **For parents and caregivers who worry about not providing the "right" food for their child.** Food is fun, food is cultural, and, for many of us, food is love and family. But most importantly, food fuels our bodies and minds. You have entered a judgment-free zone regarding your meals, snacks, and groceries. Judgments about food cause harm.
- **For parents and caregivers with trauma caused by their own childhood or experience of dieting, dislike of their own bodies, and shame experienced from living in a size-obsessed world.** We've heard from thousands of parents that while they want their children to be healthy, they do not want to put their children through what they experienced growing up: diets, calorie counting, body-shaming, guilt for wanting dessert, and even approaches such as "fat camps." We aren't yet in a bias-free world, with all body types being represented in the media, but hopefully we are heading there.

What Will You Take Away?

This book will be different from the very specific focus on obesity, weight loss, and weight management often found in other health or weight-focused books. Yes, this book will be helpful for parents who want to address their child's weight, but it's not a weight loss book. The American Academy of Pediatrics believes that weight management in children is best begun by a visit to their pediatrician and possibly by a referral for a program that specializes in obesity care or weight management.

When we want to make changes to our health habits in a world that seeks quick fixes, there can be some challenges. Families are busier than ever, and there is incredible pressure on parents to be perfect, whether that be on social media, around other caregivers, or even in their own homes. In this book, you will gain a new perspective on

- **Finding the right balance with food:** feeding our families a healthy, well-balanced meal while still having foods that are important to our history, culture, and palate
- **Reducing control around eating:** feeding our children well, without being the food police
- **Having positive weight talk:** addressing issues around weight without making our children dislike their bodies, pursue fad diets, or even talk in harmful ways about weight, all of which can lead to disordered eating
- **Removing shame or guilt:** letting go of shame and guilt around eating, despite many judgments about what we should and shouldn't be eating
- **Making activity enjoyable:** letting our children be children (eg, playing video games with their friends) and encouraging physical activity
- **Breaking cycles:** Raising our children to be healthy, while breaking the generational cycles of disliking our bodies and going on restrictive diets to lose weight
- **Prioritizing health over beauty standards:** focusing on health and not giving in to societal beauty standards and while maintaining a healthy relationship with food

Highlighting the 3 Perspectives

This book is a guide for families, based on decades of research and experience, on how to make sure your love of children comes through while trying to raise them to be happy and healthy. We are a part of the Brenner FIT (Families in Training) program, a unique interdisciplinary pediatric weight management program that is part of Wake Forest University School of Medicine, Brenner Children's Hospital, and Advocate Health, located in Winston-Salem, NC. Since our program started in 2007, our approach has changed a lot. We began trying to give families the tools to recognize what habits were unhealthy and help them replace those with healthier habits. Like many others, we recognize that no one ever chooses to have unwanted extra weight; they don't deliberately develop habits that cause unwanted weight gain or choose to have problems like diabetes or high blood pressure. There are many other things that influence a person's health, weight, and body size, nearly all of them being out of the person's control (eg, genetic makeup, food systems, income, food access, the environment). Over time, we have shifted our approach from focusing primarily on weight to empowering families to be the best they can be, recognize the pressures and stressors of life that can influence their health and well-being, and realize there is a better way for families to be happy and healthy.

As a parent or caregiver, you may have concerns about your child's weight: they may be developing high blood pressure or another weight-related health problem; you don't want them to develop one of the illnesses that runs in the family, like diabetes or heart disease; or they may be getting teased at school. You don't, however, want them to become self-conscious about their body and hurt their self-esteem by bringing these concerns up. So you feel stuck; either you say nothing and risk the problem getting worse or you run the risk of making your child feel bad by saying they need to lose weight. While changing habits can be empowering for the family, discussions of weight with your child can sometimes feel like criticism; it's a sensitive conversation for sure. If you do nothing, unwanted habits could develop, weight could get worse, and health problems could result. If you become overly focused on health and weight, you run the risk of damaging family relationships through struggles over food and activity, harming your child's self-esteem, and/or contributing to disordered eating.

In this book, we offer your family another way: **building health habits in a balanced way.** We thread the needle by incorporating lessons learned from the most current science about weight, the highest quality research on raising and feeding children, the lived experiences of people in bigger bodies, and the expertise of caring professionals involved in this work. Seems easy to do, right? We know it's not.

Throughout this book, we do our best to keep the following 3 perspectives in mind:

1. **Every family is unique.** You know your family best, so as you learn new information, think about how to apply it to your family. We present research, stories, and tips on how you as parents can lead changes in your families, and you will figure out how to fit this into your family, because no 2 families are the same. We trust you to take care of your family, and we ask you to trust us on this topic. Sometimes these strategies may seem a little different or counterintuitive to what you may think or have heard before.
2. **Nobody is perfect.** It's hard raising children, whether it was 50 years ago or present day. What worked for your parents may not work for your children, and it's easy to feel judged when things don't work out the way you intend. Many influencers on social media give the impression they live a perfect life with perfect children, and it is oh so easy. Nobody is perfect, things don't always work the first time, and change takes time. Raising children is a marathon, not a sprint, and life is about the journey, not the destination.
3. **Everyone has an opinion about health…** and weight… and nutrition…and exercise…and carbs, *especially* carbs. Unfortunately, there are many voices out there, wanting to share the secrets to healthy living. With so many manuals or self-help books out there, it can make finding the real truth difficult. A study published in the *International Journal of Behavioral Nutrition and Physical Activity* in 2024 showed that the vast majority of social media nutrition messages delivered by celebrities did not follow scientific guidelines or recommendations. Our goal with this book is to share what real research supports.

You've Got This!

Parents are often told **what** to do but don't always know **how** to do it. We wrote this book to fill a much-needed gap for parents to navigate the personal, emotional, and behavioral side of weight issues in their children. There are wonderful books that cover the *what* of weight management, nutrition, and activity in children. But this book deals with the *how*:

- ☑ *How* to talk (or sometimes NOT talk) with your children about their weight
- ☑ *How* to help them build better self-esteem about their bodies
- ☑ *How* to put new habits into place
- ☑ *How* to help children eat healthy without it causing eating disorders
- ☑ *How* to deal with pushback from children
- ☑ *How* to instill new routines without making everyone feel bad about their old ones

We provide guidance, step by step, about **how to change behaviors, develop healthy habits, and manage your child's weight in a safe and effective way.** Our goal is to support parents who want to raise their children to have balanced eating and activity habits. We know you are the expert on your family. Your opinion matters. When you aren't sure what to do next, know that you are not alone and there is a loving way to support your child.

We can show you *how.*

CHAPTER 1

Understanding Your Child's Weight

Mya and Sean have 2 children, Olivia and Kai, born 19 months apart. The siblings are very similar in the foods they like and the sports they play, and because the family is very close, the siblings enjoy participating in a lot of the same activities together. As they start elementary school, Olivia's weight increases faster than Kai's. At her annual checkup, her doctor suggests several changes for her to make: eat smaller portion sizes, avoid sodas and juice, use a smaller plate, cut back on snacking, eat more fruits and vegetables at meals, increase exercise, and decrease TV and electronics use. While not perfect, the family is very successful in implementing the recommendations. One by one, the changes suggested by the doctor are made. But Olivia continues to gain weight. Increasingly, the focus shifts to Olivia and what and how much she is eating, how much she is on her tablet, and how much exercise she gets, which leads to arguments between her and her parents. None of the focus is on Kai; he is allowed to have soda, nightly dessert, unrestricted video game time, and access to snacks whenever he is hungry. Olivia is not allowed any of these things…and she notices.

What are Mya and Sean thinking and feeling? They feel like they are responsible for Olivia gaining so much weight, like they did something wrong. They also feel bad because

Olivia is now miserable. They argue a lot more with her about food, and she feels bad about herself and is often angry with them. Mealtime is a constant battle, so now Mya and Sean tend to dread dinnertime every night. They are confused; they are doing all the "right" things, yet these don't seem to be helping her weight and are only causing frustration and arguments in the family.

What is Olivia thinking and feeling? Olivia feels angry at her parents for treating her differently, while feeling bad about herself for wanting to eat more. She remembers when things were fun, and she and Kai did things together, but now their parents seem to treat him better because he isn't big like her. She wants things to go back to normal before their parents became obsessed with her weight, before they worried about what she ate and drank and how much exercise she got.

Avoiding Weight-Focused Changes

The message is very clear: body size does *not* always reflect someone's habits and doesn't always represent their health accurately. For a child in a smaller, thinner body, do not assume they have balanced eating and activity habits. Thinner children can just as easily have picky eating or an unbalanced diet or not be getting physical activity. We also see many children in larger bodies classified as having obesity who eat very nutritious foods and are active and athletic; unfortunately, these same children are often told they need to "do better" to achieve a healthier weight, and their parent/caregiver may be made to feel ashamed watching their child continue to gain weight.

Many aspects influence a person's weight: the state where they live, the neighborhood where they grew up, genetic makeup, personality, and food access, among others. We also know that events in childhood including economic hardships, violence, and neglect can lead to stress that affects our bodies in many ways, including weight gain. Some people just naturally have larger bodies. If you look at a typical sports team, people are many different shapes and sizes, and are all "built" differently, although it is hard to know exactly what size and shape we are *supposed* to be. The important thing to focus on is being the best "us" we can be.

So let's move beyond weight; nutrition and physical activity have many other positive benefits to our children: physical activity builds strong bones, sports teach teamwork and discipline, and nutrition helps with immunity and long-term health. As our children grow older and enter adulthood, those habits have an even greater influence on their health, with balanced eating habits improving their blood pressure and cholesterol levels, exercise preventing arthritis and osteoporosis, and sound sleep habits improving their school performance. As caregivers, we want our children to develop strong lifestyle habits, so it is very important not to single children out based solely on body size but to focus on the health habits of the *entire* family.

As illustrated in the family story, focusing on the weight of a child is tricky. Making one child overly focused on their weight, and not their sibling, can lead to a lot of family conflict and make the child feel self-conscious about themselves (and can teach both children that something is "wrong" with people in bigger bodies). When more and more focus was put on Olivia, her weight increased even more (which we see happen all the time in our program). On the other hand, no restrictions were placed on Kai, as it was assumed he was healthy and OK to have soda, snacks, and desserts because he was at a lower weight. This approach made Olivia miserable (and didn't help her weight), and while Kai's weight wasn't going up, he wasn't developing very healthy habits either. Making decisions about these children based only on their body sizes wasn't working out very well!

How Much Does Extra Weight Affect Our Health?

To be clear, when we refer to "extra weight," what we *mostly* mean is extra *adipose tissue,* or *fat,* which is where we store extra energy. Sometimes this comes from taking in more energy (calories) than we burn every day, but other things can cause us to store extra energy as well—the types of foods we eat, genetic makeup, medications, and stress. For some people, extra weight might be how they are built—big bones; big muscles; tall, broad shoulders; or wide hips (and, in my family, very large heads). In general, though, when people talk about obesity, and how it can lead to health problems, they are referring to having extra or excess fat.

When it comes to this extra fat, how often does it lead to health problems? A few studies have shown that the health problems arising from excess fat, or obesity, can be attributed to the bias and discrimination people in bigger bodies face regularly, similar to the bias people face for other reasons (eg, disabilities, race, ethnicity). Discrimination and bias cause people stress, and that stress builds up over time and can cause microscopic damage to their bodies. It can cause inflammation, high blood pressure, and harm to their mental health. Over time, this stress and microscopic damage (or "wear and tear"), called *allostatic load*, can cause problems such as heart disease, diabetes, and even cancer. Also, this weight bias leads to people not wanting to even go to the doctor, which can cause them to miss out on valuable medical care. While research is ongoing, there is scientific evidence of this effect today, further supporting that we shouldn't judge or discriminate against people because of their body size or shape.

There is also an abundance of evidence that excess adipose tissue can lead to inflammation and dysfunction in our bodies. In particular, the fat around the middle of our bodies, called *visceral fat,* is noted not just to be a storage center for excess energy we have consumed but to be an active organ that releases hormones and other signals in our bodies that result in damaging inflammation, and this is one of the main culprits that can lead to diabetes, heart disease, and even some cancers. Decades of research, from large population-based and genetic studies, have clearly shown that excess adipose tissue on our bodies can cause health problems. Thus, there are important reasons for building habits that maximize our health, lower our risk for chronic disease, and, if necessary, help us lose excess body fat in safe ways. Because of the harmful effects of weight bias and its emotional impact, however, it is crucial to address weight with care and sensitivity.

The Science Behind Understanding Body Size and Shape

There has been a dramatic shift in how people understand their bodies, including the size they are. First and foremost, throw out the old thinking that our weight is all about "calories in, calories out." It is not that simple. There is so much more that determines our weight and body size. Yes, there is plenty of research that shows that certain habits, particularly related to eating, exercise, and sleep, can lead to increasing weight gain and excess body fat. As mentioned earlier, genetic makeup also has a lot of influence on body size and weight, and our habits are influenced by where we live and what we do. But also, body size does not always indicate body health. Plenty of people in bigger bodies can be healthy, and plenty of people in smaller bodies can be unhealthy. It's often assumed that if you are a "healthy weight," you can eat whatever you want. This is not true; healthy living pertains to everyone, no matter what their weight. While there have been dispute and pushback, the evidence is the evidence: whereas people with a lot of extra body fat tend to have more health conditions, the numbers on a scale are typically just a screening for potential health problems and therefore do not represent our overall health and, even more importantly, do not represent who we are as people.

What Is Body Mass Index?

Children are constantly growing and changing. Even for teenagers who may have nearly reached their adult height, their bodies are still maturing, but there are other factors to consider besides what the scale reads. For that reason, doctors use a measure of height and weight together, most commonly called the *body mass index,* or BMI. Growth charts and BMI are considered screening tools, so they are not perfect determinants of body fat, healthy or otherwise. Jaylen and Donte are 15-year-old boys whose BMI qualifies them as having obesity. Jaylen is more active and spends a lot of time weight lifting. He has more muscle mass, but his diet is limited because he has picky eating. He also tends to stay up late playing video games, averaging about only 6 hours of sleep most nights. Donte, on the other hand, is more sedentary and prefers drawing during his free time. He's always had a well-rounded diet, eating plenty of fruits, vegetables, and lean proteins. He consistently gets enough sleep and maintains a regular routine. Even though they share the same BMI, their health profiles differ. Body mass index is only one screening tool; a higher BMI indicates that a child *may* have excess body fat. It is one "data point" to consider in assessing a child's weight and health. Even as this book goes to print, many medical organizations (including the American Medical Association) question the use of BMI as the best tool for classifying someone's weight status, and the World Health Organization is working on finding a better definition for having excess body fat that may improve health. Presently, the American Academy of Pediatrics recommends that medical providers use BMI, primarily as a screening tool and as a way to follow changes over time. For the purposes of this book, we won't address it again, as the focus should be on your family, your relationships, and your habits and not solely on where your child's height and weight are on a growth chart.

Something very important to know: there is a lot that goes into determining what your child's body size will be. Again, it's not as simple as calories in, calories out. Our weight, size, shape, and amount of body fat are extremely complex, so it's nearly impossible to list all the contributors, controllers, and influences on our weight and size, assuming we know and understand all of them. A research group with the British government publishes an obesity systems map to try to represent this complexity, demonstrating how our energy balance is influenced by external and systemic factors like the media, society and culture, physiology, money, food and food systems, physical activity, the infrastructure of where we live, and the health care system. The map is so complex, it would take up half of this book!

Another way to understand the complexity of weight is through the depiction of an iceberg (Figure 1.1). Only 10% of an iceberg's mass is above water, while the rest is below the water's surface. We know that nutrition and activity habits can affect our weight, but we don't see other aspects that influence weight as well. Individual eating habits—how much, how often, and individual preferences—are all influenced by where we live, our family's and friends' habits, access to healthy or unhealthy foods, finances, the purchasing and preparing of food, and so forth. I cannot emphasize, stress, or repeat enough that our weight is not fully under our control and that there are many factors influencing it. It will never be as simple as calories in, calories out!

Chapter 1 | Understanding Your Child's Weight

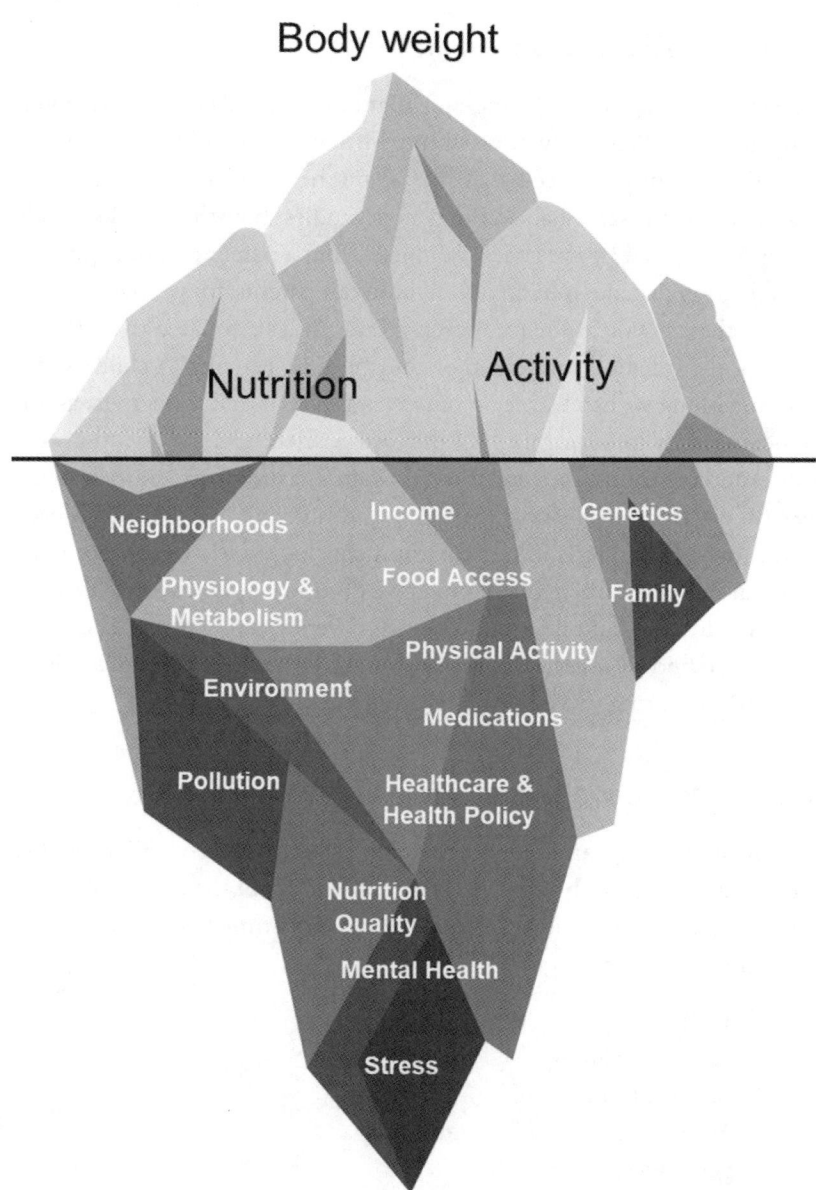

Figure 1.1. The Influences That Affect Body Weight

Genes Have a Lot to Do With It

Scientists have known for some time that our genes determine a lot about our body size. Previously, it was thought that when children are shaped like their parents, it reflects that they share the same home environment and therefore the same habits. But genetic studies show that much of body size is determined by the genes we inherit from a parent or from a unique combination of genes inherited from both our parents; for people in bigger bodies, that genetic influence is even greater, as it's estimated that 50% or more of the weight is influenced or controlled by genetics. A child's size is not something we can blame on ourselves as parents and caregivers, as it is not completely in our control. In the future, scientists may discover other causes and contributors to excess weight gain. According to an article in the *Journal of Health, Population and Nutrition,* some recent discoveries even point toward chemicals in our environment that interfere with hormone levels in our body. There is still much we don't know, but we can focus on what we do know and be open to new discoveries in the future. Therefore, we want to find balance here—ways to build habits that bring families closer without measuring success purely by weight.

We Are Where We Live

Nutrition; physical and sedentary activities; and sufficient, high-quality sleep influence a lot, but our habits are a product of the environment in which we live. For children, 5 qualities of the immediate environment can influence their weight:

1. Traffic noise
2. Safety of walking
3. Air pollution
4. Access to parks and playgrounds
5. Food access

Aside from a family packing up and moving, these factors are often beyond a child's control. The increase in weight over the past decades reflects a change in our environment (ie, food, food systems, transportation systems, technology, neighborhoods, entertainment), which directly influences our behaviors. It is important to recognize that *our habits are not a reflection of who we are as people.* Just because I do not swim does not mean I am lazy—it's because I don't have easy access to a pool! Our habits and lifestyle are heavily influenced by the environment around us, and we must take that into account when we are trying to make lifestyle and habit changes. For example, if your family does not live where there are sidewalks, scheduling a trip to a local park after school, playing a game together indoors, or dancing can be active options.

Our Bodies Like to Stay at the Same Weight

When it comes to trying to change our weight, our bodies often work against us. Our bodies fight to stay at the weight they are already at or the "set point." In 2016, a research study of a TV show where people lost an excessive amount of weight through strict diets and constant exercise showed that the contestants disrupted their metabolism in the process. When the show ended, contestants went back to their lives while still engaging in their new exercise and eating habits. Despite eating just a few more calories each day than when they were on the show, their weight went up dramatically. While on the show, the participants were eating very, very little but exercising all the time. At some point, they were losing so much weight, their body began changing to protect itself, preventing themselves from wasting away. Their bodies adapted to function on less energy, essentially decreasing their metabolism. So when they left the show, and transitioned to exercising more moderately and were eating a little more, their weight increased, even though they were still eating very little. In short, such dramatic weight loss from very strict dieting and extreme amounts of exercise wrecked their metabolism. Any slight increase in eating from their intake on the show led to weight gain. Drastic weight loss through drastic measures was *not* the way to go.

A group of scientists met in 2019 to compile decades of research about how human bodies respond to losing weight. This group estimated that for every 2 pounds of weight loss, our bodies will burn 25 less calories a day and our hunger will try to make us eat almost 100 more calories a day, to get us back to that previous weight. It can be quite difficult to change our weight, so feel free to clarify that reality when someone suggests "taking off a few pounds" as if it's something easy to do. While it can be done in safe and effective ways, it's never as simple as "eat less and move more."

> ### "Will my child's weight never change? Should we even try?"
>
> We don't mean to give you the impression that there is absolutely nothing you or your child can do about their weight. But there are some very important things to remember:
>
> - Your child is more than their weight, and there are more important things than their body size and shape: their personality, spirit, intelligence, sense of humor, and kindness, as well as the fact that they are your child and family.
> - Children come in all different shapes and sizes, and we do not have control over much of the why. This is normal and wonderful.
> - Their weight is not their health. Weight is not the only marker of their health, and there is a lot more to their health than their weight.
> - Your child's health and well-being are *way* more important than their weight and body size. Now, we recognize they may be teased or bullied about their body, and we will talk more about that later (see Chapter 3, [Not] Talking With Your Kids About Their Weight), but do not sacrifice your relationship with them, or your child's sense of self-worth, self-love, and happiness, to achieve a lower weight and smaller body size.
> - Efforts to lose weight can oftentimes be more harmful, both physically and emotionally, than being in a bigger body. I would personally rather have a happy and healthy child in a larger body than an unhappy child struggling to get to a lower weight.
> - Focusing on being healthy (see the "Reframing what healthy means" list item, on defining the concept healthy, later in this chapter), and not on being smaller or thinner, is *always* more successful and lasts longer.

> ### According to the American Academy of Pediatrics
>
> There are many advocates and activists who think that any discussions about weight with children can be harmful, particularly by increasing the risk for an eating disorder, such as anorexia or bulimia. The American Academy of Pediatrics released a report in 2016 (and reaffirmed it in 2022) about preventing obesity and eating disorders in teenagers, noting that the following factors can increase the risk for an eating disorder:
>
> - Dieting to lose weight, especially if trying to cut or burn calories (instead of focusing on improving nutrition and being active)
> - Discussing a child's weight with them, especially talking about it in the family and encouraging the child to lose weight
> - Teasing children about their weight, especially when done by family members
> - Poor body image, which isn't shocking in today's culture
>
> The report notes that eating meals together as a family protects against both eating disorders and obesity.

Helping Children (Safely) Build Healthy Habits

For decades, people have been trying to eat healthier, exercise more, manage stress, and get plenty of sleep, all in an effort to prevent poor health, chronic disease, and even early death—what you'll see referred to in medical journals as *morbidity* (illness) and *mortality* (death). There is not one "right" way to do things, and it's different for everyone. The same applies to children, but one thing we know for sure (and it's a tenet of pediatricians) is "Children are not little adults." There are some things we must do differently in children to prevent harm. What harm?

Eating disorders, fractured relationships with food, poor self-esteem and body image, malnutrition (not receiving the right vitamins and minerals for proper growth), risk for cyclic dieting into adulthood, and even relationship harm with our children. At its most basic, the family meal is a beneficial, positive thing in our families, but if we as caregivers turn into the food police, it almost always becomes a point of conflict and misery.

Following are a few reasons we must approach children differently when we are trying to change habits.

Children Are Part of Their Family and Therefore Influenced by Them

Whether your child is 4 or 17 years old, they are part of a family, and the family is the No. 1 influence on a child. So even if everyone in the family is a different size, it's important to make as many changes together as possible. Of course, children and the adults in their family spend a lot of time outside the home, and are thus influenced by work, school, and the neighborhood in which they live, but their family is still the No. 1 influence. My adult sons are still influenced by how they were raised; the habits they developed in our home as they grew up, the recipes they learned, the tastes they were exposed to, the sports and activities we did—these have all had some influence, even as they grow and change.

Family Connection Has a Big Impact

I know that seems repetitive, but we too often see families stressed when trying to make habit changes or lead healthier lives or when struggling with an illness such as diabetes. Following are some of the most common things we see causing disagreements and stress in families:

- An adult trying to get their child to play less video games and be more active
- A child who has picky eating around vegetables and is being made to feel guilty about it by others in the family

- A teenager shaming their caregiver for not cooking better dinners
- Arguments over taking a cell phone into the bedroom at night

Many families stop or give up making changes because it causes too many arguments or stress and, in the end, hurts their relationship. We don't think it's worth sacrificing family closeness for more vegetables to be served at dinner. In fact, family meals are one of the core things we want families to adopt. The more meals families eat together, the more they talk, the better they eat, the happier they are, and the better they get along. (See Chapters 5, Family Connection Is Your Greatest Strength, and 6, Small Shifts, Big Impact: Transforming How Your Family Eats, for more information on family connections and mealtimes.)

Some Children Are at Risk for Eating Disorders

Eating disorders have one of the highest mortality rates of any mental illness, are very difficult to treat, and can cause lifelong damage to physical and mental well-being. We have seen thousands of children and caregivers work toward improving their health habits and their weight. If there is tension or disagreement in the family over issues such as food, sleep, and activities, change often does not go very well. We spend a lot of time addressing tension in family relationships, especially over food management. Many adults have stories about their own childhood, including experiencing traumatic conversations with their parent or caregiver, particularly comments made to them about their weights and bodies, and being forced into damaging diets. A long-term study called Project EAT showed that when parents encouraged their teens to diet, it resulted in more eating disorders, unhealthy weight loss behaviors, greater weight gain, and low body satisfaction once the teens grew up and became parents themselves, 15 years later! Increasingly, we hear parents and other caregivers say, "I want my child to be healthy, but I don't want them disliking their body and being worried about a number on a scale like I was." There can be lifelong damage to the psyche when a person grows up worried about weight. Let's stop that cycle!

The Differences Between Disordered Eating and an Eating Disorder

Disordered Eating
- Irregular or inconsistent eating behaviors
- Skipping meals
  - Fasting: not eating for a day or more
  - Sneaking/hiding food
- Restricting what is eaten to control size or weight
  - Dieting: reducing calories to lose weight
  - Skipping food groups without a medical need to do so
  - Limiting portions
- Firm dietary rules
  - Excluding specific foods or food groups
- Ignoring hunger and fullness cues
  - Not eating even when hungry
  - Stopping eating while still hungry
- Exercising to burn calories
  - Focused exercise with a goal to "burn off" what was eaten
- Body dissatisfaction
  - Significant focus on body appearance as self-worth
  - Negative attitude toward weight and shape
- Limited or inflexible food intake
  - All-or-nothing thinking
- Compulsive eating or overeating
  - Eating very fast
  - Eating past feelings of fullness
  - Eating alone because of embarrassment

Eating Disorder
Must be diagnosed by a professional and have a significant impact on physical and mental health[a]; must occur with greater frequency and severity than disordered eating behaviors

- Anorexia nervosa: eating restriction, low body weight, fear of gaining weight, altered perception of body image
- Bulimia nervosa: binge-eating episodes of eating very large amounts and loss of control, with behaviors that compensate for what was eaten, like vomiting or laxatives; value of self that is altered by perception of appearance
- Binge-eating disorder: episodes of eating more food than typically expected, eating quickly and past fullness, often in secret and with a lack of control
- Avoidant/restrictive food intake disorder: unrelated to beliefs about appearance, feeding and eating disturbance that results in being unable to meet nutrition needs

Continued on next page

Disordered Eating	Eating Disorder

• Often socially normalized or overlooked
  ○ Behavior may fit with that of the surrounding culture.
  ○ Behavior or resulting weight loss may be praised by others even if it is out of balance.
	• Other specified feeding or eating disorder: category for eating disturbances that do not fit into other categories or meet full diagnoses of a category

[a] Consult your pediatrician to discuss any concerns.

Sources: Derived from Chaves E, Jeffrey DT, Williams DR. Disordered eating and eating disorders in pediatric obesity: assessment and next steps. *Int J Environ Res Public Health*. 2023;20(17):6638 and Dennis AB. What is the difference between disordered eating and eating disorders? National Eating Disorders Association. Accessed October 16, 2025. https://www.nationaleatingdisorders.org/what-is-the-difference-between-disordered-eating-and-eating-disorders.

Source: Adapted from American Psychiatric Association. *Diagnostic and Statistical Manual of Mental Disorders*. 5th ed text rev. American Psychiatric Association; 2022.

Affirming Our Children's Bodies

Weight and body size can be incredibly sensitive and delicate subjects, and we recommend focusing more on health and habits instead. If, however, your child brings up concerns about their body size, a health care professional expresses concerns that excess weight may be leading to health problems, or other children have teased or bullied your child about their weight, it is important to have tools to assist you in responding to your child. A discussion around weight and body size should be done carefully and gently, taking your child's age and developmental stage into account. Our job as caregivers is to affirm and love all bodies. We show appreciation for our own bodies in as many ways as we can. We can show appreciation for our children's bodies as well. We can model this acceptance of all bodies by saying what we appreciate about our own body—for example, "Glad I made it up the stairs today! Thank you, legs!" or "This shirt is my favorite, and I feel so good in it." This is drastically different from "I'm getting so old; the stairs wear me out" or "Why can't clothes look good on me? Everything makes me feel too big." We may have negative thoughts about our bodies from time to time, just like we may get angry when someone pulls out in front of us while driving. You want to set a positive example for your children by not hurling insults at or saying curse words about the driver; in the same way, if you feel something negative about your body, be careful about what you say in front of your children, as it may unintentionally teach them negative stereotypes about their own bodies.

It's also important to consider our comments about other people's bodies. When we praise a friend for losing weight, including how great they look now, there is an implication that they didn't look great before. The intention may be to praise the weight change, but the message that our children hear is that they didn't look as great with a different weight. It can send the message that being thin is the way to look better. When we notice a family member who gained weight and later comment, "Did you see how much weight Aunt Melanie had put on?" we potentially send the message that the weight gain is a concern to be discussed by others. A person's body is not our business, and we need to be careful about what we are teaching our children when we make comments about people's bodies. We can complement attire, activity, job success, creativity, sports skill, personality, or other qualities without addressing the body size/shape or change. Also, people's weight goes up and down for many different reasons, such as stress, depression, medications, or illness. I knew a person who had lost a lot of weight, so people would make very encouraging comments—when in fact she had thyroid cancer! In general, weight is a topic to approach with sensitivity. Initiating the conversation about weight with a child can unintentionally elicit feelings of rejection or criticism of their body. If they choose to bring it up, it is OK for them to discuss their concerns with you.

Every child at some point will notice how their body looks compared to others' bodies. Being sensitive, gentle, and supportive is important. If your child brings up weight with you, listen and support them. Following are suggestions on how to respond:

- **First and foremost, affirm their body as it is today.** You love your child more than anyone else on Earth and you are the one to affirm their body as it is, loving the whole child (body and all) to the moon and back.
- **Do not gaslight.** If your larger-bodied child asks if they are fat, do not tell them they are thin. Bodies come in all shapes

and sizes. You can affirm that everyone is made differently, and all bodies are wonderful. On a football team, you need people in bigger bodies to be linemen, you need fast people to play running back, and you need people with strong legs to punt the ball and kick field goals. You can affirm that their body is exactly as it is supposed to be. You can validate that they might be larger than someone else. Facts are facts and are not to be denied or lied about.

- **Comparison will cause dissatisfaction.** Size is one way of comparing. Comparison is not how to validate our worth or attractiveness. We can always find someone with a look or body feature we may strongly desire. Instead, it is important to focus on what we love about our own body and ourselves and what makes us unique.
- **Focus on positive qualities aside from their appearance:** their personality, sense of humor, character, honesty, intelligence, hard work, and kindness.
- **Tell them they are loved.** Remember that a lot of their body size and shape is not something they can change, so focusing on that is likely to do nothing but make them feel bad and frustrated. In return, tell them what they do have control over: how they treat other people, their attitude, and their participation in family activities, to name a few things.

Positive Reinforcement

There is a line from a book by Steve Maraboli that "the scale can only give you a numerical reflection of your relationship with gravity. That's it. It cannot measure beauty, talent, purpose, life force, possibility, strength, or love." We need to really internalize and live that with our children. For that reason, it's important to try to avoid the use of some particular words with children, as much as possible. Based on research about how we discuss weight and health, our experience working with thousands of families, and what they tell us about how they feel when they work with health care professionals, it is clear that words can be charged with many different meanings and affect people in various ways. Parents and other caring adults must model the right behaviors and language around children. Following are a few examples:

- **Positive body talk:** It's important for adults to model positive talk about their bodies, or even avoid talking about bodies altogether, *unless* done in a positive way. Body talk can feed into societal pressures to have an ideal body when in reality there are all body types and sizes. Some of us have long legs, short legs, wide hips, thin hips, broad shoulders, narrow shoulders, and so on. When we make comments about people's bodies, or our own bodies, it can have unintended consequences. Many children and caregivers have told us they get asked "Have you lost weight?" knowing the person is trying to say something positive, but what they may hear is "You needed to lose weight, and it looks like you finally have!" Set a positive example by avoiding body talk or by noting positive aspects of bodies, such as strength, endurance, or skill ("Look, she can roll her tongue sideways!").
- **Reframing what healthy means:** Healthy can mean different things to different people, whether it be cultural (rice is an important food in many cultures, but to someone with diabetes, it can mean extra carbohydrates and needs to be limited) or even political. With children and families, the concepts of "healthy" and "unhealthy" can lead to labeling and can influence how we feel about food. As one example, I love apples, especially the crisp, sweet, and tart Honeycrisp apples (when they are on sale), and most nutrition experts would agree that an apple is healthy. I also like a good bag of potato chips, particularly kettle-cooked salt and vinegar chips (my sons call them "stinky chips"). Again, most experts would agree that potato chips are not healthy. While there are children out there who prefer an apple over potato chips, in US culture, it's safe to say the vast majority of children would choose potato chips over an apple. If we call an apple "healthy" and deem potato chips "unhealthy" too much, particularly around younger children, they could view unhealthy foods as tasting good and healthy foods as not tasting as good.

Fast-forward to a parent trying to make changes in their home, and instead of having potato chips with family dinner, they say, "We're eating healthy tonight, so we're having broccoli"; you can imagine the look on their child's face. There is nothing wrong with a parent making changes and serving broccoli instead of potato chips, but labeling foods too much can set your children up to not like your new healthy dinner or develop a preconceived notion against what you serve. As children mature into teens, they can learn that one food is healthier than another, as well as that there is a time and place for special treats and snacks. But in raising children to be accepting of new foods, labeling the foods can often lead to pushback and resistance or, in the case of highly desirable foods like potato chips, an obsession with or fixation on them.

- **Using the words *weight, fat,* and *obesity:*** These are obviously very loaded words. Many body positivity activists have reclaimed *fat* as a personal quality and description, not a negative one, and your family may hear that term used to describe bodies. Different cultures have different ways they think of and view larger bodies. Unfortunately, most of the time when you hear these words, they will be used in negative ways. With children, we talk about how people come in all shapes and sizes, and all bodies are different. It is important we do things to take care of our bodies—for example, eating regular meals, getting enough quality sleep, and moving our bodies on a regular basis. This topic can become very complicated and is different for everyone, so we recommend taking great care in using these words. We generally prefer more neutral terms, such as *bigger bodies* or, for those struggling with a health issue, *excess weight*, and not focusing on words that can lead to undesired thoughts or behaviors.

- **Smaller bodies = healthy weight/bigger bodies = unhealthy weight:** As previously mentioned, bigger bodies are often labeled or seen as "unhealthy" and smaller bodies as "healthy" when that is not automatically true. Much has been written and researched about *metabolically healthy obesity,* where people's weights may be classified in the obesity range on a chart but the person is essentially considered healthy. I can tell you from 20 years of medical practice, I consistently see children in different-sized bodies with very similar eating and activity habits. During past summers, my son developed sleep and eating habits that were the opposite of his school-year routine. I can guarantee those habits did not support his health, despite his athletic build. If we believe someone with a smaller weight is automatically healthy and someone in a bigger body is unhealthy, that shifts our thinking to the idea that weight and body size are sole determinants of health, which is far from true.

It is also important to remember that your child's weight may or may not be affecting their health. There is a chance that extra weight could be a risk for future health issues, but you must balance that with your child's well-being. Will discussing their weight or trying to do something about it do more harm than good? Will a diet and exercise plan make your child miserable, affect your relationship, and make them feel bad about themselves? Are the changes you make ones that will last, or that your child will keep doing for years, or ones that your child will do just a few months to lose some pounds? Nearly all strict diet and exercise plans will eventually end, and the weight will often return. Focus less on weight, and more on habits, family, relationships, and a love of one's body, the enjoyment of food, and the appreciation of movement, in order to launch your child into adulthood with sound and solid habits that can last a lifetime. We conducted a project with our adult weight management colleagues and found that families can actually be closer by changing habits together, in a family-friendly way that is not focused on weight. Spending more time together in positive ways is beneficial; planning a meal together, without a focus on calories, has a better outcome on a family than telling a child they can't have second helpings of their potatoes because potatoes are high in carbs and will cause more weight gain.

Our message here can be told by using 2 old sayings:

1. **A watched pot never boils.** Focusing too much on a child's weight and their habits may see short-term changes, but those are unlikely to last and the child will probably fall back into the old "diet and exercise" routine that has not made much of a

Chapter 1 | Understanding Your Child's Weight

difference in our world. Take a longer-term approach to weight and health.

2. **Don't miss the forest for the trees.** Too much focus on a child's weight or body size, and on the immediate habits of diet and exercise, will miss the broader things, such as your family, long-term health habits, relationships, and well-being. While details are important, which we will talk more about in this book, *how* we do things related to our family habits can be just as important as *what* we do, if not more.

So where are Mya and Sean and their children now? One night at dinner, Olivia asked for second helpings of mashed potatoes. Sean said, "No, you've had enough." Olivia protested that her brother already had 3 servings and didn't eat his vegetables. Afterward, Sean and Mya realized how unhappy their dinners had become since they began focusing on Olivia's weight. They talked with their children's pediatrician and made some changes in how they navigated mealtime:

- Focus was taken off Olivia and her weight.
- Focus was put on the family schedule: meal and snack times, homework times, free time, and family time.
- Children were included in decision-making, both in meals and in free time and family time. This gave them some say in the routine, but their parents still remained the parents (eg, if Olivia and Kai said they wanted to have donuts for the evening vegetable, the parents got to say no).
- Everyone followed the schedule, including the parents.

Initially, there was some pushback from Kai. He still wanted unlimited access to snacks instead of snacks only after school, but within a few weeks, he adjusted to the new routine. The children enjoyed keeping their parents in line too, pointing out when Sean snacked on things while dinner was being cooked. Most importantly, there was no pressure on Olivia, and everyone felt like a part of the family. Olivia's weight gain slowed down, and she continued to grow taller. Even more importantly, her relationships improved not only with food but with her body and with her parents. While Kai was considered to have a healthy weight, his eating habits also improved, and while he still enjoyed playing video games, he had limits on how much he could play every day, as he understood what the rules were and followed them. Mya and Sean no longer felt like "failures" with their parenting (To be clear, they were never failures!), and disagreements over food and video games all but disappeared.

CHAPTER 2

Parenting Through Structure and Love

Keisha is a single mom to 8-year-old Jasmine, who was a large child right from birth (9 pounds). It seems like everyone in Keisha's life has advice about how to slow down Jasmine's weight gain and help her find a "normal" weight, including her aunt, grandmother, teachers at school, and doctor. They advise her to serve Jasmine smaller portions, eliminate junk food, provide healthy snacks, not allow second helpings of meat, serve more fruits and vegetables, avoid desserts, and cut down on screen time. Keisha does her best to manage all this advice, but it's difficult as a single mother; some days, Keisha is exhausted after a long day at work, so it's easier to stop at their favorite fast-food restaurant for dinner, which features an indoor playground that Jasmine loves. They both order what they want, and Keisha loves watching Jasmine go down the indoor slides. She worries about her daughter's weight, though, because Jasmine's grandmother has type 2 diabetes and Keisha struggles with her own weight. She read about how both these things are influenced by genetic makeup and put Jasmine at risk of experiencing them as well. Also, children are starting to tease Jasmine. Eventually, Keisha starts following the advice given to her, in particular, stopping their fast-food outings.

Within a week of making these changes, such as offering no second helpings of her meats, only fruit for snacks and dessert, smaller portions for dinner, and high-fiber, whole-grain cereal for breakfast, everything changes, but not in the way Keisha has hoped. From the moment Keisha picks Jasmine up from her after-school program, Jasmine keeps saying she feels hungry. She eats her meals fast, and once, she actually vomited. She sneaks food at school and steals from other children's cubbies. She even starts calling herself fat!

What is Keisha thinking and feeling? She regrets making these changes. None of these changes feel good for her or her daughter. Jasmine's weight isn't improving, and Keisha dislikes how dinnertime has become a constant battle. Keisha has rich memories of her childhood family meals with everyone eating at the table, talking about their day and laughing. It hurts that nothing is working out like she had hoped. She feels frustrated that this new lifestyle seems to be backfiring, and Jasmine's vomiting scares her. Other questions and thoughts running through her head are

Because of Jasmine's fast eating and vomiting, I should double down and limit food even more.

Maybe something is wrong with Jasmine. Could she have bulimia? Does she have a stomach problem?

I need to explain to Jasmine that I am making changes because I love her, and in the long run, they will pay off.

I can teach her about calories, so she knows to choose things that are low in calories.

What is Jasmine thinking and feeling? Jasmine is very confused about all the drastic changes happening. She loves her weekly fast-food dinner with her mom, but it was taken away entirely. She does not understand why her mom did that and wonders if her mom is upset with her or thinks she is fat. She thinks her mom is being mean for not allowing her to eat what she wants and can't stand it when her mom tells her she's had enough to eat. All this change hurts her feelings a lot and is eroding her self-confidence.

The Most Important Influences

Parenting is the toughest job you'll ever love! And this may be obvious already, but the family and the home in which you are raising your child are *the most* important influences on your child, their health, and their development. Now, much of what lies outside your home you may not have control over, but you are the window to the world for your child. The good news is that children are resilient. If you surround them with love, you are giving them the best chance to thrive. Don't stress!

When it comes to living a healthy life, the most common things we hear from parents and caregivers are "I tell him to eat less candy and more vegetables" or "I keep reminding her to go outside and play." When it comes to some old-fashioned food adages or sayings, we do not agree with the Clean Plate Club or "No dessert until you finish your vegetables," as science and experience tell us those often backfire. Implementing these sayings can result in children disliking foods even more, and forcing children to eat their veggies before earning dessert oftentimes results in them disliking veggies and becoming obsessed with sweets. As far as telling your children to do something healthy and expecting it to happen, I'm here to tell you that "Do as I say, not as I do" doesn't work either! No matter what the age of your child, telling them to do something related to health will not yield long-term positive results. **To make change happen, it needs to be a combination of**

- Showing them the change by modeling the behaviors you want them to develop
- Setting them up for success by having a structure and schedule that point them in the direction you want them to go

These 2 things will prevent the undesired side effect of pressure and restriction (we call it the **P & R Coin;** more on that in the P & R Coin: Pressure and Restriction section later in this chapter) where we try to control what they do too tightly.

A Scientific Approach to Parenting

Diana Baumrind was a developmental psychologist who conducted research on parenting behavior in the 1960s and categorized parenting styles based on her observations of preschool children's behavior patterns. Through observing children in different settings and by interviewing parents, she identified parenting styles and how they influenced a child's development. In the 1980s, Eleanor Maccoby and John Martin, researchers at Stanford University, later expanded on Baumrind's work. Their work is still being used today to better understand how to best parent children, and elements of this work can be found in many modern parenting books. Collectively, this work focused on 2 important components, or dimensions, of parenting, in particular, the finding that *how* caregivers do things can be just as important as *what* they do.

- **Warmth, acceptance, support:** It's called many different things, but a key part of parenting comes down to the **love** a child feels from their parent. Ideally, all parents love their children, but children may not always feel or sense that love, so when we do things as a parent, even things like correction, punishment, or discipline, we want to make sure we do so from a place of warmth and love.
- **Control, strictness, demandingness:** Parenting with **structure** and discipline in the home is another key component of raising children. Contained within this is that a child knows the rules of the home, and the parent is in charge of these rules and expects the child will follow them, while recognizing that children often learn through trial and error and may not meet parental expectations their first, second, or even third time.

But taking a scientific approach to parenting doesn't stop here. Parenting with warmth, acceptance, and support can easily be misinterpreted as spoiling a child and not doing anything to upset them, while parenting with control, strictness, and demandingness can be misinterpreted as running a regimented household with 100% obedience. If only it was that simple; there are never clear and easy rules when you are a parent. Baumrind, Maccoby, and Martin's work led to expansion of the following 2 parenting dimensions to balance warmth and control:

		Demandingness: structure and control	
		High	Low
Warmth and support	High	**Authoritative** Clear rules and boundaries, but affectionate and supportive	**Permissive** Few rules and boundaries, but affectionate and supportive
	Low	**Authoritarian** Clear rules and boundaries, less supportive and nurturing	**Neglectful** Few rules and boundaries, less supportive and nurturing

Source: Baumrind D. Current patterns of parental authority. *Dev Psychol.* 1971;4(1, pt 2):1–103.

Derived from Maccoby EE, Martin JA. Socialization in the context of the family: parent-child interaction. In: Hetherington EM, ed. *Socialization, Personality, and Social Development.* 4th ed. Wiley; 1983:1–101. Mussen PH, ed. *Handbook of Child Psychology;* vol 4.

While there are many other theories of parenting, authoritative parenting is thought by parenting experts to be the ideal approach and has been well studied in the nutrition and obesity fields. This parenting approach is not universal and may not apply to all cultures or situations, but authoritative parenting is an effective approach to raising children. Children raised in those households are typically happier and self-confident as well as show more independence, perform better in school, and have better relationships with friends and families. Children raised in authoritarian, permissive, or neglectful parenting households, on the other hand, generally encounter more struggles with their behavior and education, although this possibility depends on cultural, social, economic, and educational factors, as well as the personalities and characteristics of the family members. When it comes to concerns about weight in children, children raised in authoritarian households tend to have greater weight gain over time, while authoritative households see the lowest weight gain in children and raise children who are less likely to have excess weight.

Parenting is about balancing discipline in the home, implementing reasonable rules that children can understand and respect, and maintaining a structure, a schedule, and expectations, with expressions of warmth and love. Strict disciplinarian approaches, as in authoritarian parenting, often result in children not feeling loved, feeling insecure, and having negative self-esteem.

How Do You Parent Around a Child's Habits?

Be it preparing meals, encouraging physical activity, establishing strong sleep habits, or doing well in school, parenting in a way that has your family adhering to clear rules, schedule, and structure tends to work the best. Now, we aren't saying to run your household like a strict military unit—it's your family after all. So this is what the message comes down to: structure and love. There are several other ways to say it: schedule and warmth, rules and affection, strict but loving. The point is that children thrive when they know what to expect, what the rules are, what is coming next, and when each "what" occurs with support, love, and affection.

It is inherent in every parent or caregiver that they approach parenting with a set of rules and structures and with love for their children, but with the everyday stressors of life, sometimes that daily schedule falls apart and we don't always show our children the warmth and affection we feel for them. So bringing those things back to the forefront in our everyday lives is the key to raising healthy and happy children. If you decide "I want to change what my family is eating" or "We aren't active enough—we're on our tablets too much!" and want to make a change, that is a great start. We want you to be successful, but we also don't want to cause division or arguments in the home, which are something we observe and work through every day in our clinic. Adults may become frustrated when they can't make a change in their family's habits, children feel bad because their parents make comments about what they are eating, or one member of the family is singled out because of their habits or their weight. Why incorporate healthy habits if they only cause families to be unhappy with each other or make someone feel bad about themselves? Making changes should occur together with minimal arguments or feelings of failure. Using the Structure and Love approach is a great way to do that, but it's important to keep a few things in mind:

- **Children's behavior is often in reaction to something.** Think back to when your children were babies and began crying. You tried to figure out why: Was their diaper wet? Were they hungry? Were they tired? Did they need to be held? You went through the checklist until you found the reason they were crying. Even as children grow older, oftentimes they act out in response to something. In the P & R Coin: Pressure and Restriction section later in this chapter, we explain that children sneak food when they feel restricted. Sneaking is a natural response, especially with younger children, to restrictive messages about food and their weight. About 99% of the time, we find that when children sneak food, it's because they are being told to eat less, they feel self-conscious about what they are eating, or a certain food (typically a favorite snack or treat) has been made off-limits. When you see your child reacting to a change you make, try to figure out what your child may be experiencing, or what they may be thinking and feeling (like we share in the beginning chapter stories), and consider how using the Structure and Love approach can help.

- **Maturity level matters.** We know children have different understandings at different ages, but sometimes we forget that. With school, friends, and activities, our children spend a lot of time outside our home and away from us, so we eventually want them to make healthy choices themselves. I am here to tell you…they likely won't. They are still learning after all! Children are constantly growing up and maturing, and at certain ages, they aren't cognitively mature enough to do certain things without guidance or supervision. An analogy I often use in the clinic is that I wouldn't let an 8-year-old drive a car, so I wouldn't expect them to pick a balanced meal of nutritious food when their favorite snack chips are also available. Their frustrating lack of interest in changing health habits is totally normal and natural.

- **Every child is different.** This sounds cliché, but I often tell myself this with my own children. My 2 boys are as different as night and day: looks, personality, likes, dislikes, and even their accents (my older son has lived a good part of his life in Wisconsin, while the other has in North Carolina). How we parent one child is completely different from how we parent the other. That doesn't mean the Structure and Love approach won't work for both, but *how* that is implemented can differ. One child needs to hear "I love you" often and is physically affectionate, hugging us hello and goodbye; the other child is less physically affectionate and prefers one-on-one time with each parent individually. For grandparents who are the caregivers, this can be an important lesson, as raising children in today's world is drastically different from when they were parents with young children in the home, and while some things are eternal (children needing to feel secure and loved), the challenges are different (eg, internet, smartphones).

Health Habit Guidelines

At what age can you expect children to take responsibility for their health habits or to make changes on their own? It can vary widely, depending on the situation and the child. We generally adhere to the following guidelines in our clinic:

6 years and younger: Making household change is 100% on the adults! While children this age may be interested in their bodies, including wanting to be strong or fast, they generally won't understand concepts of prevention or health, at least not in the way adults do. They are kids—let them be kids!

7 to 12 years old: Children in this age range begin to understand more, but we would not expect them to make changes on their own. They can understand and learn concepts around nutrition, exercise, and sleep, but this understanding won't translate over to them making habit changes. They are much more influenced by their parents, their peers, and their home environment and schedule.

13 years and older: Teenagers! Adolescents! Young adults! Teens are more influenced by friends and their environment, and parental influence, while still important, starts to wane a bit. It's tempting as a caregiver to try to assert that influence again, but that can also lead to conflict if done too sternly or directly. As teens develop more independence, they will practice setting their own structure step by step. Older teens can take responsibility for making changes some of the time on their own with less and less assistance.

The P & R Coin: Pressure and Restriction

Decades of research in child nutrition and behavior have identified 2 concepts parents or caregivers apply hoping for one result and creating an opposite result: **pressure and restriction,** representing 2 sides of the same coin. They are different, but they are related and can end with the same result. This P & R Coin may sound a bit like reverse psychology at times, but with growing and developing children, pressure and restriction are powerful forces that can have the opposite of the intended effect or, in a sense, backfire.

Pressure: If we pressure our children into eating (eg, "Eat your vegetables," "Eat this plum"), it usually has the opposite effect (ie, not wanting to eat their vegetables, not liking the plum). When a child is forced to eat something, it may become a negative experience. An example we hear every day is a child being told no dessert unless they eat all their vegetables. We know this usually results in children loving sweets and not liking vegetables. Pressure to eat a food → negative feelings around the food → not liking that food.

Restriction is the flip side of pressure and has the opposite of the intended effect. The most common restriction is limiting second helpings of certain foods during a meal. Most of us may be familiar with the direction "You haven't eaten your veggies, so no seconds of spaghetti." Think about a holiday or special event, like a birthday or a cultural tradition that occurs only once or twice a year where children indulge in their favorite foods. They really, really like it because it's special and rare! When we set limits on the foods that are offered, it can make them more alluring and more desirable. Or if an offering is something that isn't that rare, like spaghetti, but we tell them not to have too much of it, it can make them want it even more. Even at snack time, limiting amounts of the snack (ie, allowing half a banana with 1 tablespoon peanut butter) can cause overfocus on the limited food and often leads to sneaking food. Restriction also leads to overeating at times.

> ### No Misinterpretation Here
>
> The P & R Coin can easily be misinterpreted as "Give children only the food they want, and never encourage them to try anything new" or "Let children eat as much as they want, when they want." Neither is the intent. The P & R Coin is something that is used when families try to make changes in children's health habits—for example, limiting how much they eat, serving smaller portion sizes, pressuring to eat fruits and vegetables, making electronic time dependent on the amount they exercise, and forcing sports or exercise on a child who doesn't want to participate. Unfortunately, these are the common suggestions parents are told by friends and family, and they often lead to the opposite result. Telling a child to eat less of a food will cause them to want it even more, which can lead to sneaking; similarly, telling a child to eat more of a food they don't enjoy will often make them dislike it even more, which can lead to avoidance and non-preference of that food. Staying away from pressure and restriction, but using the authoritative parenting tenets, like having structure, rules, boundaries, and expectations in a loving environment, can help parents achieve their family's health habit goals.

One of the best known approaches to feeding your family in an authoritative manner was developed by Ellyn Satter, MS, RD, CICSW, BCD. From her experience as a dietitian and therapist working with children who faced eating disorders and dieting failures, she developed the Satter Feeding Dynamics Model and the Satter Eating Competence Model. Supported by decades of research by scientists such as Leann Birch and others, she wrote the Satter Division of Responsibility in Feeding, which provided a framework for raising a child to have a healthy relationship with eating. We have found this model particularly useful for all ages and have applied it in our practice around physical activity as well. In this model, caregivers are responsible for *what* food is being served, *when* it is being served, and *where* it is being served. For parents, the model stops there. It lifts the responsibility of the adult having to be the food police, or monitoring calorie for calorie what their child is eating, because as the P & R Coin demonstrates, becoming too involved will often end up backfiring.

In turn, your child is responsible for *if* they are going to eat and *how much* they are going to eat. When I was in my pediatric training in the early 2000s, a very experienced pediatrician told me that over a month's time, a child's body will tell them what they need. Some days, they will eat a lot; other days, they won't eat as much. Some days, they will eat a lot of protein; other days, they will eat a lot of fruits and vegetables. Both my boys eat like that. Even to this day as young adults, their appetites and preferences vary day-to-day and week-to-week.

Dr Clara Davis: Changing How We Look at Children's Diets

A fascinating, legendary study from the 1920s and 1930s by Dr Clara Davis details how giving 15 children, who were all malnourished, the opportunity to feed themselves from a wide variety of foods allowed them to grow to be healthy and well nourished, even though they all ate differently. It's as if each child knew what their body needed!

Unfortunately, much of those data are lost, as only one paper and one presentation exist from it. At the time, it was thought there was a right and wrong way to feed children, and for children who were not growing or eating well, a strict, doctor-prescribed diet was the only answer. Dr Davis turned this thinking on its head by allowing children to pick from 33 different foods offered to them. For the 15 children she studied, they had 15 different individual, unique eating patterns! And all the children thrived on their own self-selected diets. The foods being offered were very nutritious (fruit, vegetables, whole grains, and cooked meats, including liver, kidney, and brains!); however, the key was not to force a prescribed healthy diet on the children but to let them choose from the selections offered.

Continued on next page

> While this was some time ago, and many details are lost to history, it significantly changed the thinking on how caregivers should feed their children.
>
> **Source:** Strauss S. Clara M. Davis and the wisdom of letting children choose their own diets. *CMAJ.* 2006;175(10):1199–1201.

Putting Structure and Love Into Place

Using the Structure and Love approach in your own home takes time and patience, but once it's in place, parents tell us it's less stressful, gives them more time to focus on each other during meals, and helps mealtime be an enjoyable time again. Instead of watching how much your children eat of a certain food (ie, being the food police), focus on trusting them with their eating.

Children listen closely to the words we use around food. What we say can affect how they think and feel about their hunger and fullness and whether they trust their own bodies. Here are some simple swaps for common phrases that help create a more positive and supportive environment while still setting kind and helpful limits.

Common Phrase	New Phrase	Why It's More Effective
"Take 3 more bites of chicken before you get more mac and cheese."	"You can stop when you want."	Encourages your child to learn to trust their own internal fullness cues
"Eat your vegetables. They are good for you."	"Would you like some vegetables with your meal?" or "Here are some veggies if you'd like to try them."	Offers vegetables without pressure or moralizing
"Should you really be eating that?"	"It's not time to eat right now, but you can have that when it is."	Sets boundaries without judgment

Common Phrase	New Phrase	Why It's More Effective
"Finish the rest of your meal and you can have dessert."	"It is OK if you can't eat everything."	Removes pressure and encourages them to listen to their internal fullness cues
"You cannot possibly still be hungry! You ate more than I did."	"It's fine to have more. Once dinner is over, the kitchen is closed."	Respects hunger cues while setting limits
"You've had enough sweets today."	"We had dessert at lunch today. We can have that tomorrow."	Sets limits without moralizing
"You need to make healthier decisions."	"How about we have cheese and crackers today and chips tomorrow? It's good for our bodies to have variety."	Encourages variety without shaming
"Don't be picky. You have to try at least one bite."	"It's OK not to like everything. Would you like to try a bite or not?"	Encourages exposure and autonomy without shame

Children thrive in knowing their surroundings, being comfortable and familiar with their environment, and knowing the limits of what they can and can't do. Most children will figure out the rules, but they will feel much more comfortable if these rules are laid out for them ahead of time and they then have the opportunity to practice, stumble, and fall, with trial and error. Know that it may take a few times for your children to fully embrace a revised schedule, and they may push the boundaries, but if they are corrected or reminded in a loving fashion, they will eventually pick it up. If you want the best for your child, implementing some structure into the daily routine will allow your child to thrive, teach them the habits you want of them, and provide the best way to raise them in a healthy and happy manner.

> **"But I don't want to be so strict!"**
>
> Think of the best teacher you ever had—not just your favorite teacher but the one you liked and respected and who taught you well. In addition to being creative in how they taught, they were effective in what they did, and you learned a lot. Maybe it's because of the structure they had in their classroom. Sometimes they may have even been strict, but you likely felt they cared for you and wanted you to succeed. How much would students learn if there weren't rules about raising their hand, asking one question at a time, or adhering to start and end times to class? If the teacher was harsh and made you feel bad, you likely would not label them as a favorite teacher, right? (And while a fun-loving teacher with no class rules would be a blast to have, you likely wouldn't learn that much.) Applying some type of structure in your home, when trying to raise children with healthy habits or when trying to change some habits, is key and can be just as effective.

Implementing structure within the home and setting clear rules and expectations can be hard for families that struggle with a set schedule. We don't expect anyone to be perfect, but in time, families can make the schedule work for them as they learn what works and what doesn't. The next few chapters will cover this topic in more detail, but let's briefly review how structures and schedules can help with making habit changes.

> ### "Does this apply to sleep too?"
>
> Whether for an infant or an older adult struggling with insomnia, a good night's sleep is all about structure and schedule. For children, it comes down to quantity and quality (ie, making sure that they get enough and that it is good). Experts believe most sleep problems can be improved or even cured with strong sleep hygiene, most of which is based on having an appropriate schedule at bedtime and maintaining a good sleep environment. This pertains directly to sleep quality; we know that when our children sleep with phones in their rooms or have other electronics on right before bed or during the night, they don't sleep as well. And poor sleep not only makes them tired but disrupts their internal systems and can affect their health. Poor sleep can lead to high blood pressure, disrupted hunger cycles, and fatigue. Setting rules and a schedule for sleep that are appropriate will go a long way. For most children, this involves having a nightly routine to decompress from the day, distancing from electronics and media, preparing for the next day, and setting up their bed or room for a successful night of sleep—quiet, dark, and electronics-free.
>
> Love can be applied to sleep. For younger children, it may be reading a book with them or lying in bed and discussing your day together. For older children, it may be helping them get ready for the next day, packing a lunch, or preparing breakfast ahead of time. For teens, even if they don't show appreciation for it, it may be asking about their day, telling them you love them, asking if they need anything before bed, and ending the day with a positive interaction.

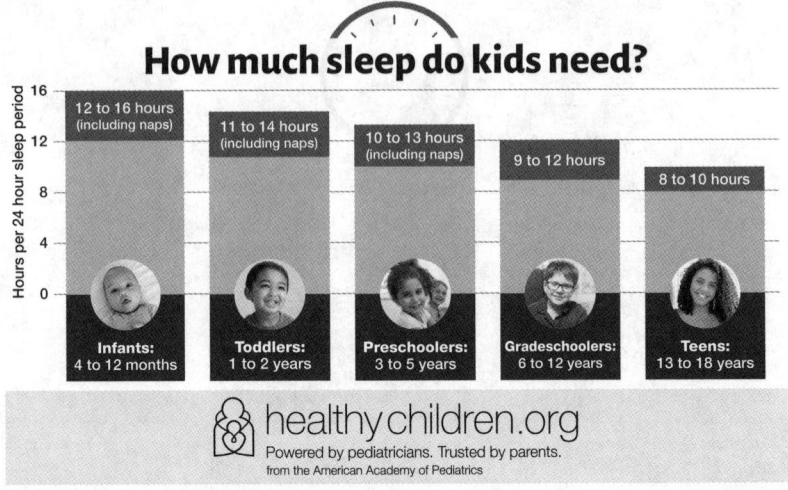

*The American Academy of Pediatrics (AAP) has issued a Statement of Endorsement supporting these guidelines from the American Academy of Sleep Medicine (AASM).

Source: Paruthi S, Brooks LJ, D'Ambrosio C, Hall W, Kotagal S, Lloyd RM, Malow B, Maski K, Nichols C, Quan SF, Rosen CL, Troester MM, Wise MS. Recommended Amount of Sleep for Pediatric Populations: A Statement of the American Academy of Sleep Medicine. *J Clin Sleep Med*. 2016 May 25. pii: ic-00158016. PubMed PMID: 27250809.

But How Does the Structure and Love Approach Apply to Activity?

Activity can mean a lot of different things to different families, such as physical activity, exercise, sports, games, sedentary (sitting) activity, video games, and electronic time. For our purposes, we'll lump this into 2 categories: physical activity and sedentary activity. We know for some people, this isn't much of a struggle, whereas for others, it is a *huge* challenge, so it is difficult to know where everyone falls. For most of us, our work, school, and family schedules can lead us to not being very active, so we have to constantly work around that. For lots of children, sports (team and individual) are the primary outlet for physical activity. Over time, that changes: as children become older, they may focus on 1 or 2 sports or lose interest in sports altogether, particularly as sports get more competitive, more expensive, and more time consuming. Nearly all children will be exposed to and enjoy some form of electronic entertainment, whether that is social media, video games, internet searching, or virtual reality (by the time this book is published, something new will probably be out). For some children, this can be overwhelming or be their primary form of entertainment, even a social outlet through multiplayer online video games.

Both physical and sedentary activities can be points of conflict for children. For physical activity, if they begin to play sports less often or lose interest in sports, we see their parents pressure them to exercise more. Many children and teens won't find a lot of traditional exercise, such as running, walking, weight lifting, going to the gym, or swimming laps, to be all that fun or entertaining. They are naturally reluctant to do things that are not considered fun and resort to other activities, often those that are sedentary. Whether the activity is exercising or eating broccoli, pressuring them will often backfire.

By implementing *love,* we do not judge the activities children enjoy doing, such as playing video games. Physical and sedentary activities are not all or none! Children can enjoy video games, but like with any recreational activity, there are limits to how often they can play them. Spending time together, in both sedentary and physical activities, can also be an expression of love and a way to grow closer. *Structure* can be applied by setting reasonable limits on some of these sedentary activities. If parents create structure around media and electronics use (no phones or tablets at the table or within an hour of bedtime), there may be some initial arguments as rules and limits are instituted, but it will eventually eliminate the daily fights about screen time use. By still allowing these sedentary activities with limits, you can help balance their days with physical activities. Scheduling time to be electronics-free becomes part of the house rules and routine. These are *not* easy parenting tasks to navigate, we know, but in time, they can provide your child with the opportunity to engage in things they and their friends enjoy but include limits so they have time for other pursuits. See Chapter 7, Parenting Through Exercise and Physical Activity, for more information.

Structure, Love, and...Eating?

There are many aspects to children and their appetites that structure and love work well for. One of the best things you can do for your family is to have more meals together. Whether your family is eating at a restaurant, ordering takeout, or cooking a meal at home, spending more time together improves many aspects of your family habits and your health (see Chapter 5, Family Connection Is Your Greatest Strength). Eating meals together is an opportunity for connection. As a parent or caregiver, when you feed your child or teen, it is nurturing them. This is a chance to pair the nurture of the meal with the nurture of connection. Take time to talk about the day, go over "highs and lows" (see the "Encourage people to talk" list item later in this section), and express gratitude. There are many benefits to having family meals; be sure to tune in to your children's interests at this time and take advantage of the conversation. Your children learn how to manage life from hearing stories about how you manage home or work issues. Maybe you spent an hour on the phone trying to get a prescription filled and covered by insurance; share that frustration. Maybe a coworker helped you complete an important task, and you appreciated their support. Stories are ways of sharing with our children how we build relationships and are thus an avenue for them to learn about relationships with others. This time over a meal together is incredibly valuable.

Focus on each other (love) and use the mealtime as a period during which to check in with each other and talk about your day. Most children (yes, even teenagers) feel loved when their family is spending time together, their parents are talking with and listening to them, and a feeling of closeness results from this time together. Make it a mealtime (structure), as best as your schedule allows, by designating the time the meal is being served and finding a place to serve everyone, be it the dining room table or even a blanket spread on the living room floor for a picnic. Don't feel the need to push your children to try a food, but continue to offer the food without pressure. Pediatricians and other feeding experts have recommended offering foods over and over, without pressure to try them. The more children become familiar with the food, the more likely they are to eventually try it. An old saying is that parents have to offer a specific food 15 or more times before children will accept it. When children try a new food, it can be fun to talk about the process and to even describe aspects of the food, but be careful that children don't feel the pressure to eat a lot of it or have to like it, as that can also backfire. There is a fine line between encouraging a child to try a new food and pressuring them; a parent may not intend to pressure their child, but they still may, so keep the meal positive, the encouragement light, and the pressure to a minimum or not at all. Implement rules such as eating at the table with the rest of the family, but avoid telling children what they can and can't eat from what is being served.

The approach we've developed over the years for parents to put structure and love into place is outlined in the following ways:

- **Involve the entire family.** The saying "Teamwork makes the dream work" or "There's no I in team" truly applies when making health behavior changes at home. Children are more likely to embrace new habits when they feel supported by the whole family and not singled out. When everyone works together, it creates a sense of unity and encouragement that helps children feel safe, included, and motivated to follow the plan. In our clinic, we consistently see better outcomes when families work together and maintain consistent expectations for everyone. This shared effort builds connection, accountability, motivation, and common goals, all of which increase the chances of long-term success.
- **Create a routine and practice consistency.** When children know the schedule, they can plan ahead and know when the next meal or snack is. As each new school year started, we would often write down the bedtime until it was routine to head off arguments about what time to get ready for bed. Find out who has after-school activities (eg, practice, tutoring, work), who will be around in the evenings, and who is present for dinner each night and record all of those as well. Allow for flexibility, as things can come up, and schedules become busy. Place the schedule somewhere where everyone can see it, then build your week, including dinner plans, around that. In posting the schedule for the week, the family is aware of the daily ebbs and flows and of what everyone is involved in. During times in my own family where we were busy, and not spending a lot of time together, my sons sometimes didn't even know where I was. Having a schedule can help provide children with all the family information.
- **Plan ahead for meals and snacks.** Lots of families may have dinner together, but because of work and school schedules, breakfast and snack times can vary. If breakfast times vary in

your household, make sure you have food ready and available. We have found that while most people might schedule dinner at a certain time, or even budget time to cook a meal or pick up takeout, they don't schedule time to go grocery shopping. As part of your weekly meal planning, make sure to schedule time to go to the grocery store and to prepare meals.

- **Remove pressure and restriction (P & R Coin).** To support your child's eating, try removing comments that pressure your child to eat their vegetables or that restrict them by encouraging them to eat less food. Caregivers can demonstrate this change by providing regular meal and snack times and not judging how their child eats from the food that is provided. If your child eats more than you would expect, or is avoiding certain foods, that is OK. Pressuring or restricting can lead to shame and guilt about food. When you remove this stress, your child can better tune in to their hunger and fullness cues and explore new foods at their own pace, which lays the groundwork for a healthy relationship with eating that lasts into adulthood.
- **Model the behaviors you want to see in your children.** If you don't want your children to have snacks before dinner, don't snack yourself. Try the new foods being served with dinner. Plan a balanced meal with several food groups to include everything on it. Schedule time for yourself to be active, and make sure you get enough sleep as well, without taking your phone into your room at night.
- **Make time to connect.** For families new to eating meals or doing activities together, it can help to have a list of things to talk about. My family would often engage in "highs and lows": conversations about the good things that happened to us during the day and the not-so-good things. This can serve so many purposes. In addition to improving communication, it can take the pressure off a member in the family who has picky eating, or it can give a family a new focus besides the habit of watching TV or using a smartphone during the meal.
- **Schedule activities together.** Show your interest in something they enjoy and do it together. Take turns on who gets to choose

the activity, which can defuse the arguments or negotiating that can occur in families. You can try their chosen activity, and they can try yours. Pick a legitimate activity you enjoy, like a hike or a sport, or going to see a play—that was always mine!

Once your family is in a routine of having a schedule around meals, snacks, and activities, you'll notice that your children start to follow that schedule more. Knowing when snack time is and when dinner starts provides reassurance for children, because they know when meals are offered, making it one less thing for them to navigate and one less thing for you to worry about. It also provides the opportunity for parents to be a role model, possibly introduce new foods, try a new recipe, or even experiment. Children are used to coming to the meal at the designated time and are typically hungry, as they have learned to have snacks during snack time and not graze throughout the day. Coming to the meal hungry means they can be more open to new foods, particularly when served alongside a familiar one. For video games, media, and electronics, they understand they will get to play, and have access to these fun activities, but know ahead of time when they need to stop. Fights about bedtime will decrease, because it's the rule and schedule of the house, but don't be surprised when they try to test the limits again in the future. Making a change is not always easy, but in time, your family can establish clear routines and expectations for everyone.

How did structure and love turn out for Keisha and Jasmine?
As Keisha waited to see a stomach specialist about Jasmine's vomiting, she came to me to address her daughter's increasing weight. She shared how she was trying to slow Jasmine's eating and explained all the changes she was making to improve her weight. Jasmine had never experienced stomach problems before. At first, Keisha made attempts to set up a schedule for meals, but then she realized she was putting a lot of pressure on her daughter. She was so scared about Jasmine's weight gain, and the risk for diabetes, that she wasn't seeing how her fear made Jasmine feel. Ultimately,

Keisha had become an authoritarian parent, controlling how much Jasmine ate, putting pressure on her at every turn to eat more fruits and veggies, and restricting her access to the foods she enjoyed. It would be easy to see their weekly visit to the fast-food restaurant as "permissive," but it was only once a week. More importantly, it was a special, relaxed bonding time for them to spend together.

After explaining authoritative parenting to Keisha, including the idea of structure and love, and how Jasmine would not be able to make healthy food choices on her own, Keisha eased up a bit, reinstating their weekly fast-food dinner. We worked to reframe this meal as a family night together. They ate at the table, turned electronics off, and enjoyed their food without stress. Both Jasmine and Keisha benefited from this weekly habit and made it a family routine. Keisha also instituted a meal schedule where Jasmine could eat until full during the meal, and when the meal was done, the kitchen was closed. She stopped making comments about how much or what to eat and instead enjoyed the time with her daughter. Keisha was so focused on adhering to the meal schedule, and enjoying the lack of stress over trying to control the food Jasmine ate, that she didn't even realize Jasmine's eating pace had slowed down and the vomiting had stopped completely.

By lifting the pressure she placed on Jasmine around eating, and keeping their fast-food date night, Jasmine no longer ate as fast as she could or snuck food. The vomiting stopped, the stress dropped, and they were both happier. Over time, this change set up Keisha to make further changes. They scheduled time to take hikes on weekends when the weather was good, and when fast-food Wednesday was reinstituted, they found more time to play together on the playground. Keisha felt more confident trying a new recipe or including a variety of foods in their meals. While there was not a short-term improvement seen in Jasmine's weight, there was great improvement in their meal schedule, Jasmine's eating pace, and their relationship. This set them up for long-term improvement in their habits, and they were much happier as a family.

CHAPTER 3

(Not) Talking With Your Kids About Their Weight

Manuel is the father of two. He saw his doctor for a checkup and was found to have high cholesterol levels. His doctor suggested cutting back on eating red meat, so Manuel and his wife, Rhonda, decided to leave the ground beef out of their family's favorite spaghetti recipe and replace it with marinara sauce after announcing to the family that they were going to start eating healthier by trying a healthier spaghetti sauce. This became a big deal in the family, because that was the children's favorite meal, and every Tuesday was Spaghetti Night!

This "new" spaghetti has become very unpopular with their 2 children, who dislike it and refuse to eat it. Suddenly, the best night of the week for the family is now filled with bickering about the spaghetti and requests such as "Can't Dad have his own spaghetti, and we get to have ours?"

What are the parents thinking and feeling? They feel frustrated because they think the new meatless spaghetti tastes fine. Why do their children dislike it so much? Can't they understand this change is important not only for their dad's health but for the whole family too? Spaghetti Night is now ruined! This change is very small, it is important for their health, and they both think the change doesn't affect the taste of the spaghetti that much. Manuel and Rhonda both

> feel disappointed that this makes their children so upset and adds stress to a special mealtime.
> **What are the children thinking and feeling?** Why does their dad's cholesterol have to mess up their favorite meal? Can't he just eat something different? Why weren't they asked their thoughts first about changing Spaghetti Night?

Talking About the Word *Healthy*

It's natural to teach our children valuable lessons, help them understand why we do what we do, and foster dialogue about values that are important to our family. So it's natural to talk with our children about eating healthy meals, doing physical activity to strengthen our bodies, and getting plenty of sleep. But, oh, if it was just that simple!

When it comes to food talk, some studies show that labeling foods "healthy" and "unhealthy" can have the opposite outcome with how children think the food will taste; more specifically, they may think that healthy food will taste bad and that unhealthy food will taste good. One study from the *Health Psychology* journal featured my favorite apple—the Honeycrisp—and data showed that calling it "healthy" led people to choose it less often than if it had been given a subtler message, such as being represented with the heart-healthy symbol. Children, especially those who are younger, are not often invested in a food being healthy; it's not a selling point to them. Sure, a Popeye-like message of spinach making you strong can help a little, but in the long run, calling a food "healthy" will not pull them in. Children may eat a food you encourage them to, but they may be doing so to please you, not to feed their hunger. The opposite can be true as well: portraying food too much in a negative way, calling it "unhealthy" or "bad" for your body, can turn it into a forbidden fruit, likely making them want it even more. Imagine a meal where you push your child to eat their broccoli, calling it "healthy," but then talk negatively about the unhealthy brownie and ice cream after the meal. To a young child, this may teach them that unhealthy is tasty and healthy is not tasty. To be clear, I *love* broccoli—it's one of my favorite foods—but to a child, if broccoli and brownies are placed side by side, nearly every child will choose the brownies! Even teens, who are able to reason at a higher level, often make food decisions based not on health but rather on the level of enjoyment. By definition, teens have a feeling of invincibility and will not think about health issues over the long term in the way adults tend to do.

Defining What Healthy Means

Think about what healthy means to you. Then think of your favorite comfort food, snack, or indulgent food. Chances are, it is not considered healthy by nutritional standards. We often label tasty foods as "unhealthy"/ "junk food" or foods we can eat on "cheat days." I absolutely love southern-style biscuits and gravy, and while I know it's not nutritious, it's something I enjoy sporadically. But good gracious, it tastes delicious. My children also love this meal, and they see it as a treat we have periodically, so we celebrate it, as it is linked to their grandparents, great-grandparents (my grandfather called it *sawmill gravy*), and culture. It's like a birthday cake; it has meaning to our family and we have it for a special occasion.

For my coauthor Dara, macaroni and cheese is associated with every meal eaten at her grandmother's, as it was her beloved grandmother's delicious recipe. Thus, it is not only tasty but nostalgic. When it comes to our favorite foods, particularly those that hold important meaning for us, we want to keep them as part of our lives. Some dishes or recipes may even add variety, comfort, cultural meaning, and history to our lives. They will remain important to us, whether they are healthy or not.

Who defines what healthy looks like? Currently, there is a revolution in nutrition research, with many old ideas being disproven as well as new ones emerging. We must recognize that studying nutrition and health is *very* difficult, because every year, there are new scientific tools that lead to new discoveries. What is healthy for one person may not be healthy for another, and what works for one person (eg, low carbs, high protein) may not work for another (ie, high carbs, whole grains). Some cultures maintain physical health with a low-fat diet, while others do well with high protein. As your children go out into the world and are interpreting different messages, it can become even more confusing. For children being raised in a family from China, India, or the Philippines, their family may include rice in meals on a regular basis because of preference, cost, and cultural importance. Imagine how confusing it would be for that child to then hear from a health care professional that rice is high in carbohydrates and can cause diabetes! The same would be true with some families from Mexico or Central America where tortillas are a staple in meals. In the thousands of families we have cared for over the past 20 years, we see the confusion that comes from trying to apply a "one size fits all" approach to nutrition. While there are some universal truths of foods and activity (too much salt, sugar, and saturated fat and too many ultra-processed foods can be harmful, and more lean proteins, whole grains, and fruits and vegetables can be helpful; moving is more helpful than sitting), applying strict rules or offering simple recommendations to everyone is not helpful. You have permission to enjoy foods from your family's culture without guilt and to teach your children to rely on and prepare the same foods.

Avoid Labeling Foods

When serving foods to your family, you don't need to label them "good" and "bad" or "healthy" and "unhealthy." Instead, adopt a more neutral approach when talking about them. Food is food, and it is important to enjoy all different types and textures and flavors. As children become older and start asking more questions, it's OK to talk about how some foods, like biscuits and gravy, are foods we eat less often because they have more saturated fat. They are also part of your family's traditions. My ancestors ate them to give their bodies energy for working hard on the farm all day. Today, we don't need that much extra energy, so eating them all the time wouldn't be the best for our heart health. They are still, however, offered and enjoyed periodically without guilt.

In the same way, you don't need to label common breakfast options such as oatmeal and fruit salad as "healthy" either. As children move into their preteen and teenage years, they may ask why oatmeal and fruit are served most days of the week instead of the family favorite of biscuits and gravy. Being careful not to sound "preachy" or pressuring, it's fine for you to answer these questions about why you have one specific food over another and why having a balanced breakfast of oatmeal and fruit will be better for your health, such as improving cholesterol or blood pressure. Be careful not to link these choices to weight, particularly for younger children, so they don't equate food with numbers on a scale.

Children learn a lot from their parents and caregivers and home life, but there is a typical part of growing up where children may push back or resist when pressure is applied to them. This can be especially true with food, particularly if foods are labeled as "bad" or "unhealthy" but they are a favorite food of the child. If a healthy food is served in place of a highly desired, favorite food, the contrast can be made worse, and your child may resist even more. Think back to Manuel and his family; they loved their spaghetti, but then it was changed to include a "healthier spaghetti sauce." If your child has fruit snacks packed in their lunch every day and then these are substituted for an orange because "It's better for you," imagine how your child now perceives the fruit snacks and orange. We may hope our children are mature enough to understand the point of the change, but often they aren't thinking past "I want fruit snacks!"

As a parent, to increase our child's acceptance, we do well not to label foods one way or the other. As the parent and caregiver, you are responsible for your family's eating, so make this food part of the family routine that your children become accustomed to. For parents planning a change in their own eating habits, we typically want everyone on board, on the same page, and ready to work together. For families, we couldn't agree more. We love the Family Meeting, where family members meet to talk about different things, plan for the week, and openly express their feelings (see the "Family Meeting" box later in this section). But when it comes to discussing our bodies, weight, and individual health, care must be taken or we run the potential of causing harm, inducing hurt feelings, damaging self-esteem, and/or creating an obsession about the appearance of our bodies. In the end, the 2 most powerful ways to influence your child's eating patterns are

1. **Repeated exposure:** The more familiar a child is with a food, the more likely they are to eat it. Many children and adults say they don't like a food but have never tried it. Greater familiarity and exposure (Remember offering a food 15 or more times to a child?) increases their chances of accepting and eating it. Even involving children in preparing a food (eg, washing, cutting, or cooking it) can be an effective way to introduce them to the food and potentially have them eat it. In all of us, there is a tendency to fear new or unfamiliar foods (a bowl of

fried crickets is not something I would make at home, but it is commonly eaten in Thailand), so the more familiarity with a food, the more likely we are to try it. I was never a big fan of beans (of any kind) growing up, but trying them in different ways, in different settings, I started to tolerate them. When I learned how to cook them, and became very familiar with the different kinds, I began to really like them and even crave them at times. I imagine if I lived in an area where fried crickets are common, and became more familiar with the dish, I could eventually learn to eat and possibly enjoy them.

2. **Modeling:** Children watch us, and while there can be times they push back and do the opposite, they will generally develop the same eating patterns as their family. While some of this influence is related to repeated exposure (if an adult doesn't like cucumbers, they probably won't serve this food very often, decreasing their child's exposure to it), *how* a caregiver, an adult, or a family member talks about a food will likely influence how their child sees it as well. Aside from labeling foods as "healthy" and "unhealthy," if a parent repeatedly calls a food "gross," it's not surprising when a child also labels it that way, even if they haven't tried it.

The Family Meeting

Family meetings serve as a regular time for family members to check in with each other. They model problem-solving, communication and cooperation, and organization. As families become busy, it can be hard to keep track of everyone and stay connected. Family meetings can be a great relationship builder for your family, allowing everyone to be on the same page, learn what one another is doing, and simply spend positive time together. While it can be difficult to get into the routine, the benefit to you as a caregiver, and to your entire family, is immense. When looking to implement the Family Meeting in your house, consider the following tips:

- **Prepare.** Find a time that works for the entire family to meet. Meetings don't have to be long, and you can modify the time depending on your children's ages. It can even be as short as 10 minutes or less, where you focus on your family. In a busy family, even just a few minutes focused solely on your family can be beneficial. Set the date and time and where you plan to meet. A restaurant or public place might be too distracting, so make sure it's in a convenient location that is comfortable for everyone. Meetings can be set as weekly, biweekly, or monthly or scheduled as needed, although creating the routine is recommended. Weekly meetings can be an effective way to start as the family gets used to them and then moved to monthly if needed.
- **Plan.** The first time you try a Family Meeting, start with something simple and fun, like planning the next family vacation; that's a good way to break the ice and get everyone used to meeting. For the next meeting, make a simple agenda and write it down. This ensures you cover everything that is needed and gives everyone the opportunity to put something on there. Agenda items could include tackling one part of the calendar, such as the new school year, and what time everyone arrives home from school. Slowly, add more agenda items, such as
  - List all activities for everyone in the coming week or month, including what big events are coming up, school schedules, tests, and homework and after-school responsibilities. You can even divide lists between school, work, and family, organizing in the manner that works best for your family.
  - Meal planning can involve putting dates on the calendar for having meals together or making sure you have what is needed for breakfast, lunch, and snacks for most preferences.
  - Children can add agenda items for family discussion such as wanting to stay up later on weekends or having a sleepover for their birthday party.

  You don't have to cover everything on the agenda, particularly if it's not urgent. Items on the Family Meeting

agenda can be carried over to the next meeting. When planning the meeting, everyone can see what is coming up, which can be a good way to learn how to plan and prioritize.
- **Conduct.** Keep the meeting fun and lighthearted, so no one dreads it. Encourage, but don't force or pressure, everyone's participation. You can rotate responsibilities between family members to set the standard that this meeting is for the family and not just for the parents (although a shared load will make your job as a parent much easier). Take turns having someone "run the meeting" by going through the agenda, someone taking notes or putting things on the calendar, and, if needed, someone acting as timekeeper, making sure everyone has time to speak and go through the agenda. My family made use of a dry-erase board and family calendar that hung on the refrigerator. Family members can put things on the agenda that they want to discuss. Suggest something yourself, so children can get a sense of what purpose this component serves. Don't let this be a time to air sensitive topics or to focus anger at another family member.

Don't stress about the family meetings. Your family will likely go through periods of not needing them or become too busy to have one scheduled. If you aren't in the routine of having them, don't panic; just start them back up when possible and use them to benefit your family. They are there to help and not to add another responsibility. Use them when they are helpful, and come back to them as needed to help your family function and get along better. If they don't seem to be helping, rework them; change the agenda, the duration, the frequency, and the topics you want to discuss at meetings. The goal is to help children feel like they are part of the family and have a say in how things are run, to facilitate communication between family members, and to lower stress levels by having people be on the same page (ie, they are following the same rules and schedule).

Talking About Weight (Hint: Don't)

So you are concerned about your child's weight. How do you bring it up and discuss it? In short, don't. That might sound direct, and it is! But discussing weight and health with your children can be a sensitive conversation for the following reasons:

- **Weight is not something we have a lot of control over.**
  It is true that our diet, activity level, and sleep patterns absolutely can affect our weight. But as mentioned in Chapter 1, Understanding Your Child's Weight, much of our weight, body size, and overall shape is affected by genetic makeup and the environment we grow up in. Parents can control their home environment by setting a predictable schedule for when eating will happen and setting limits on screen time, but they don't always have control over the neighborhoods, cities, or states they live in. Because there is much about body and weight that is not under our control, we recommend not focusing on things that are influenced greatly by factors outside our control.
- **No matter how careful we are, words about weight and bodies can hurt.** In just the past few years, more research supports what we have seen for nearly 20 years: conversations between caregivers and children around weight, and even about health when the focus is weight loss, do not go well. They can cause tension, negatively affect parent-child relationships, and unintentionally make children feel bad about themselves. As we noted in previous chapters, when children feel bad about themselves, it can harm many aspects of their life and can often result in the opposite effect we were aiming for. Several recent studies have shown that children in larger bodies do not prefer many of the conversations caregivers have about their weight. Let's respect our children's voices and their ability to guide how we discuss weight.
  - Teens overall prefer their parents to talk about weight less often; if their parents do talk about it, they prefer them to be more compassionate and respectful, as the conversation makes them feel insecure, embarrassed, or hurt.

- If parents make negative comments about their child's weight, it can harm their child's health and sense of well-being.
- Parents and caregivers really want advice on how to talk about issues related to weight, including how to do so in a positive way. Children want their parents to be supportive without criticizing their weight or pressuring them, to be more sensitive and encouraging, and to focus more on health and not their weight.

- **Comments about other bodies can also hurt.** Be a role model by keeping away from discussions on shape, fat, or size. Model specific practices on this as well, not making negative comments about your own body or the bodies of others. There is a lot of research on eating disorders and weight stigma, including the damage and harm that can occur when people make comments about bodies. When we comment that another adult looks good after losing weight, we send the potential message that the person didn't look as good when carrying the additional weight. We imply that the goal is to be smaller in order to be beautiful. We cannot have our children believe this faulty cultural norm. It is harmful. Many of us grew up in this environment and know the pain of hearing comments about our own body size when we gained or lost weight.

What is going on with our bodies is our own business. There could be instances where someone in a larger body is losing weight because of cancer treatment, stress, an eating disorder, or an undiagnosed illness, so their weight loss may not be something to admire but be a cause for concern. As caregivers, we can model more of a desired behavior by holding off on sharing weight comments about others and about ourselves. Instead, talk about why your new shirt is your favorite because it feels soft and comfortable, and do not comment on the jeans that you think make you "look fat."

Hidden Meanings of the Word *Health*

In our extensive experience working with families, we have heard people use phrases and words that have been referred to as "veiled health talk." Many activists, eating disorder specialists, and parents note that while we *say* we focus on health, these phrases and words can be used as a way to criticize, judge, or discuss weight. For example, a caregiver might say, "We're going to get fit together" or "Let's start eating clean." While these comments may seem encouraging, they can send a subtle message to children that their bodies are not acceptable as they are and potentially foster negative body image from a young age. This is particularly pertinent to the topic of prevention. For children in larger bodies or with obesity, there is concern that excess adipose tissue on their bodies will cause problems later on.

Others feel this type of talk is a way to try to force children to be in "right-sized" bodies, believing that if children feel bad about their weight or fear health problems, it will spur changes to happen, but we know it won't! Shame is not a helpful motivator. Even worse, it can lead to eating disorders. Author Virginia Sole-Smith wrote an entire book on this topic titled *Fat Talk,* reporting on the social pressures on children involving weight and body size.

This is a very complicated topic, and we may never know if there is a "correct" answer to this: Will these children stay healthy even with extra fat on their bodies, or will that excess weight slowly cause health problems? There is likely truth to both sides; regardless, we don't want too much health and weight talk to unintentionally cause problems between a parent and their child or, worse, make children feel bad about themselves.

Many people, including parents, caregivers, health care professionals, and children, want to talk more about health instead of weight but can easily turn the focus back to weight.

> Children easily recognize when we substitute the word *health* for *weight* (eg, "He's got to start exercising more! I'm worried about his *health*" or "I'm fine with how he looks, but I'm worried about his *health,* so that is why I'm reminding him not to eat too much at dinner"). We've seen this in the work we do in communities, where we talk a lot about changing habits and improving health, but we end up focusing only on the numbers on a scale (ie, the weight). We know this comes from a place of love and concern, as we don't want our children to be teased or to develop a health problem that can be exacerbated by excess fat on their bodies, but it can quickly make our children feel bad about themselves or feel blamed for something that is largely out of their control. Focus on strengths and support. When we feel supported and valued, we are more likely to engage in desired behavior change.

Words Have Meaning and Impact

Many people have taken control over the description of their bodies and have pushed back over the negative descriptions of bigger bodies. Fat activists and fat liberationists have reclaimed some of this control, pushing back against the ideal body and, as we discussed in Chapter 1, Understanding Your Child's Weight, the assumption that a smaller body is healthier than a larger body, which is not always accurate. The work of the Rudd Center for Food Policy and Health at the University of Connecticut and other researchers has shown that words we think would motivate caregivers and children to make changes in fact do the opposite, resulting in negative feelings about themselves.

An *International Journal of Obesity* study with teenagers who were pursuing weight management provided some guidance around words they prefer to use about weight. Instead of *obese, chubby,* or *fat,* they preferred *weight, overweight,* and *heavy,* with some girls preferring the word *curvy.* The teens said they felt sad and embarrassed when parents used words such as *fat, big, unhealthy weight, obese,* and *weight problem.* Similar research was almost identical with the words doctors used, with parents and children not liking the words *fat* and *obese*. There is belief that these negative words may motivate children to change, but they actually don't. In fact, use of such words hurts, embarrasses, and shames them!

In the book *Positive Discipline: The Classic Guide to Helping Children Develop Self-Discipline, Responsibility, Cooperation, and Problem-Solving Skills*, Dr Jane Nelson states, "Where did we ever get the crazy idea that in order to make children do better, first we have to make them feel worse? Think of the last time you felt humiliated or treated unfairly. Did you feel like cooperating or doing better?"

Addressing a Necessary Conversation

A conversation may be needed if your child or teen is

- Beginning a medical program or seeing a medical specialist related to weight
- Being bullied about weight
- Asking questions about their body or weight

Otherwise, the conversation is not needed. Instead, focus on empowering your child to love their body or focus on habits that can benefit the whole family.

It's clear that children would prefer to talk about their favorite social media personality or influencer over their health or their weight. So when weight discussions are warranted, they need to be handled with care and the times you talk about weight need to be limited. Provide honesty and support and empowerment when talking. They need to hear more affirmations about their body than frank conversations about weight.

Always Consider Your Choice of Words

Think about what you want your children and teens to hear you say about health and weight. Notice times when there is a critical comment about weight. How could you change what is being said so that size isn't criticized? When parents are frustrated about having to buy new clothes a few months into the school year because a child outgrows what they have, it can be easy to fuss and blame the child for growing so fast. This causes stress. Avoid hurtful comments by taking a breath to calm down so the frustration isn't placed on your child. Refrain from any negative comments about your child or teen's body completely. Another piece of advice is to never weigh your child at home. This can be part of a medical exam as needed but can lead to harm at home. It overfocuses on the scale and the weight, which don't take into account a child's height and typical growth (when children grow taller, they naturally go up in weight because of muscle and bone growth, but this change could easily be interpreted negatively). Additionally, decide if a conversation needs to happen about weight. Why do we think it is needed at this time? If the goal is to make sure your child knows they are in a larger body and needs to eat less—whoa! Switch gears and (metaphorically) bite your tongue.

So What Should Conversations Focus On?

Sometimes conversations about weight will be inevitable. We know this parenting task is a lot and it's complicated. Following are some tips on how parents or caregivers can navigate conversations or issues related to weight, health, and habits:

- **Normalize discussion in small, ongoing conversations.**
    - Focus on small conversations rather than one big talk.
    - Discuss topics such as growth and health in everyday moments.
    - Don't feel pressure to cover everything at once.
- **Find times when it is natural to talk about weight.**
    - When a child comments about their own size or someone else's size.
    - When others, including a health care professional, mention your child's weight.
    - When weight-related topics appear on TV or social media
    - When there has been bullying about weight.

- **Listen without offering advice.**
  - If your child seems withdrawn or upset, ask if it's a good time to talk. If not, offer another time.
  - If your child is upset about a weight issue and shares this with you, offer your support, not a diet or a trainer.
  - Explore their feelings and offer empathy. You don't have to solve the problem or try to offer a quick fix.
  - Consider involving a pediatrician or counselor if needed.
- **Use questions to encourage your child to talk.**
  - Use open-ended questions such as "What do you think about...?" instead of "Are you worried about...?"
- **Avoid pressuring your child to talk.**
  - Let your child know that they can talk to you about weight or size if and when they are ready.
  - Avoid pushing them to talk if they choose not to.
- **Affirm your child's body just as it is.** It is most important that children hear adults affirm that they do not have to be a certain shape or size to be loved or valued. Their body is wonderful just as it is.
  - Tell your child "You are the only you, and your body is the only one like it in the world; it's doing its job well!"

Addressing Teasing and Bullying

While children may know they weigh more than other children their age, or have a bigger body, their interpretation of that can vary depending on their age and developmental status. There is a painful time when children become aware that they don't match what society describes as an "ideal" body size/weight or when other children begin to tease them about their body. That can be difficult to navigate as caregivers, and our first instinct is to protect them from this harm.

- **Listen to your gut and try to sense what your child needs at that time.** That may mean listening about what happened, discussing what happened, or just being there for them.
- **Let them know it is not OK to be bullied.** If they were called "fat" or some variation of it, affirm that this is not OK. It

doesn't matter what the words were; it matters how the words made them feel. Any form of bullying or teasing about weight and body size is wrong, period.

Only after your child or teen has had time to be reassured that they are OK and to calm down, decide on a follow-up plan.

Moving Forward With Action
Bullying is not solely the child or teen's job to correct. If this occurred in a school or another setting, it must be reported to a trusted adult such as a teacher, social worker, counselor, or principal. You or your child can report this, but let your child know this choice can be whatever makes them the most comfortable. Some children don't want to be the one to go to a teacher or principal to discuss the matter, and others don't want their parents involved; empower them to choose. If this was outside a school setting, take it to the other child's parent or caregiver or to the leaders of the organization in which it occurred, such as a sports league the children are part of. In other public settings, where you may not know the people or the organization, approach the reporting carefully, with safety in mind; you can figure out people to contact or report at a later time.

Do not promise to help your child lose weight. This implies they deserved to be teased because they are in a larger body. This is false. It is also important not to deny your child's body. If the teasing involved the word *fat*, it will not help to say, "You are not fat." Your child is aware of their size in comparison to their peers' size. Consider saying, "All bodies are wonderful, and we are supposed to be all different sizes. No one should be called names about their body." There is a tendency to want to make changes in health habits to get children to a lower weight or smaller body so they aren't teased or bullied, and that is absolutely understandable. It's going to take a long time before we rid the world of weight-based teasing, and we often think we can change ourselves before we can change the world. But you must weigh the potential harm that can occur in tactics such as strict diets, pressure to eat less, and more body talk in the home. There is a small likelihood that these things will improve your child's weight and stop the bullying in a short amount of time. Further, it is known that other children teasing your child about their weight will often change what they are bullying about, switching from weight to hair color to height to clothes. Improving the behavior of a child who bullies involves teaching that child more appropriate behavior as well as looking into factors contributing to that child's less appropriate behavior.

We should always address teasing and bullying, and schools and caregivers must stand up and stop this behavior. The quandary of how to respond when your child or teen is upset about their body hits hard. Knowing what to do day-to-day will give you more confidence as you navigate a sensitive and often painful topic. You cannot prevent harm in all circumstances. You can make sure you support your child in the following ways:

- **Listen to your child talk** about what happened, in their words, without strong reactions. Give them space to share and express their feelings without interrupting. Always take name-calling, teasing, or other bullying seriously.
- **Name the feelings** you hear to demonstrate that you understand how your child is feeling: "You sound scared of this student" or "You seem embarrassed about what she is saying to you."
- **If there is bullying, *act*!** Your child can tell a staff member at school what happened if that is where the bullying has occurred. If the child doesn't want to tell the staff, a parent will need to call the school and speak with a trusted adult such as a teacher, counselor, social worker, or principal. Schools know how to manage bullying, and we see them being very responsive to bullying concerns. If the bullying happens at another activity, contact the appropriate leaders to address your concerns. You can always figure out later with whom to discuss the matter if there is uncertainty. If teasing or bullying occurs in the home, by a family member or friend, speak with them immediately.
- **Create your own affirmation.** An affirmation is a phrase that you can repeat easily and often and has meaning for you. An affirmation to repeat to your child could be "I love you just as you are. Your body is just right." Consider what message

you want to provide your child or teen when they share that they are upset about their body. Our tendency is to try to fix the problem. We may even promise to help them lose weight so bullying will end or so they will feel happy. Remember that these myths are easy to reinforce but they are not true. Losing weight does not end bullying or automatically make us feel happy. Our job is to support our children and affirm them just as they are. They are not the person at fault in a bullying situation. They do not have to change to deserve freedom from bullying. Repeat your affirmation when your teen approaches you for support. While they may become tired of the repetition, they will also know that you love them unconditionally and are saying it out loud when they need it the most. All bodies are wonderful, and all bodies are different. Children need to be reassured that all bodies are wonderful and that comments about people's bodies or weight can be hurtful.

As a reminder regarding these sensitive conversations you will have with your child, be gentle and respectful as you proceed with caution with the following guidelines:

- **Keep the focus on health, not weight.** While we strongly believe that our focus on eating, activity, and sleep should be centered on *health,* be careful that focusing on this is not another way of focusing on *weight,* as mentioned in the "Hidden Meanings of the Word *Health*" box earlier in this chapter. For younger children, discussions on health are probably not needed; figure out the change you want to make in your family and do it, without the discussion. With older children, this can also be done, but they are much more likely to pick up on the change. Be open and honest about why you are making a change but without the specific goal of weight change (eg, "Sleep is important to us. We perform better at work and school with enough sleep, so we're going to turn electronics off a bit earlier"). This can be brought up during a Family Meeting if larger, family-level changes are needed, such as packing lunches the night before, changing morning

routines and schedules, splitting up shopping trips, or assigning new chores to children.
- **Actions speak louder than words.** As we will talk about in Chapter 5, Family Connection Is Your Greatest Strength, family affirmation and support are key. Take action by setting up schedules or eating together at the table (or counter or coffee table) or planning regular weekend walks. You can tell family members you are going to the gym and even include them in planning for it (eg, securing child care, scheduling time to go). If there is a discussion as to why the change is needed, it can be an appropriate time to discuss the health reasons, such as "Doing exercises there helps with my back pain" or "To build strong muscles and bones" and even a reason as simple as "It's a boost to my mood!" Modeling this behavior to others in the family will have more of an impact than talking about it. The reason for going is specific to how you feel, not to calorie-burning, which can lead to disordered eating behavior.
- **Help your child feel confident about their body.** Focus on what their body does versus how they look. Send the message that you want your child to grow and be healthy, not look a certain way. Teach children to respect all bodies, whatever size or ability. Talk with them about unrealistic images of bodies on social media and TV.

The Person Who Does the Bullying

What if the person who is bullying is not another child but a sibling, grandparent, or coach? This is a very difficult situation to handle. Bullying in any form is unacceptable, and when this manifests in a family member, it can be just as harmful. Weight bias and weight talk within families can increase risks of eating disorders and causes emotional harm. Family members and friends may be making comments they think are helpful (ie, "I want them to be aware," "They should know how extra weight affects their health," "I want to motivate them"), but these will only do harm. The comments may even be masked as a joke but still hurt deeply. Or the bullying may involve insults or name-calling. As you would approach a teacher or school administrator about another child who bullies, it is best to address the family member, coach, or adult directly. Situations can vary, so use your best judgment of how direct to be and how likely the chances are of educating them on the harm they may be causing. It's up to you on how much to share or how direct you want to be. Examples of things to say include

- "We are aware of his weight. We'd prefer to keep this between us and him, and we ask that you not say anything about it."
- "Please don't discuss her body anymore."
- "A child's weight, and even an adult's weight, is more about genetics, biology, and where they live. He doesn't have a lot of control over his weight, just like he doesn't with his hair or eye color. We like to focus on being healthy and not on a certain body size."
- "Name-calling of any kind is not acceptable and it must stop."

Discussions can also lead to action, and visits with family members can be stopped if they are damaging to your child. You may choose to leave an event early or not return to a harmful situation. Consider saying "The words being used to describe my child are hurtful. I think the joking is meant to be in fun, but it is not fun for my family. I need for the name-calling to stop." Remember that most people don't understand how complex a person's body is. It is essential when they are a family member, or someone your child interacts with regularly, to put a stop to bullying or harmful comments.

What about Rhonda, Manuel, and Spaghetti Night? Manuel had to balance the ruin of Spaghetti Night with his need to cut back on saturated fat to improve his cholesterol levels. So he and his wife discussed with the children how they were switching to ground turkey breast for Spaghetti Night. Both children were thrilled. They were happy with the ground turkey instead of only marinara sauce, and Manuel was happy with the leaner meat choice. Manuel and Rhonda both thought, "What if we had made the change without making such a big deal about it in the first place?" Labeling it as "healthy" drew more attention to it and, in retrospect, removed the protein portion of the meal, which was a *huge* change. In the end, Spaghetti Night was saved!

CHAPTER 4

Talking With Children About *Your* Health Changes

Jordan's mom, Beverly, had gastric bypass surgery and lost a lot of weight a few years ago. This has greatly improved her health. She cut back on several of her medications. She also loves the praise she receives for her new weight. She has changed so much that friends don't even recognize her. She feels better, has more energy, and enjoys wearing smaller clothes. At times, however, she finds herself dissatisfied with her body. When looking in the mirror, she still wants a smaller waist and more toned arms. When she tries on new clothes, she asks her teen what they think: "How do I look? Do my arms look fat? Does this hide my belly?"

Jordan also struggles with body image and doesn't know what to tell their mother. They think their mother is too focused on appearance and what others think. Jordan knows because they feel this way as well. Jordan wears clothes that are unique and is exploring how to express their identity with different outfits and hairstyles. When Jordan dresses and asks their mother how they look, their mother comments that the black T-shirt is "slimming" or the boots make their legs look "longer and thinner." Jordan understands these comments are attempts at being positive but also feels like the comments are critical. Jordan also hears their mother when she praises a friend for losing weight and "looking great" or gossips with a friend about a neighbor who "gained back all that weight" after a diet. Beverly's focus on her body's appearance, linking her own self-satisfaction with being smaller, and her comments about Jordan's body have led to Jordan feeling unhappy in their body as well. Both Beverly and Jordan want to love their bodies but are struggling to get there.

What is Beverly thinking and feeling? She has lost a lot of weight and feels so good; thus, she assumes Jordan will also feel good. Beverly thinks back to childhood meals and remembers the daily pressure to clean her plate, not wasting food, and the times when food was unaffordable and very limited. These memories provide a feeling of relief that she can provide enough food for Jordan. The two of them don't have a lot, but they don't worry about having what they need. Beverly learned from limited food access to eat when food was available, even if she wasn't hungry. She connects this fear about scarcity to her overfocus on food and weight gain. Beverly feels encouraged that she and Jordan can support each other to get their bodies more toned.

What is Jordan thinking and feeling? These physical appearances aren't that important to them, and they wish their mom would quit bringing the topic up. Jordan thinks their mom sees them as fat and ugly and needs to lose weight like she has. They don't understand why their mom is so obsessed with new clothes and appearance. Jordan resents their mother's expectation of them having to be a certain size to be attractive or happy. Jordan's body image is complicated and they deeply feel their mother's judgment of weight gain or loss in others. And they feel like a disappointment to their mother.

Changes Involve the Entire Family

A friend and colleague who is a doctor in adult medicine made this comment to me several years ago: "My patients with kids have a harder time with their health than those who don't have kids!" I pointed out to her that the "patients with kids" she was talking about were some of the same people I saw in my clinic—parents! As pediatricians, we probably talk with caregivers as much as we talk with children. It was a funny paradigm shift for my adult medicine colleague to realize her patients were also parenting!

As caregivers for our families, we would sacrifice anything for our children, often to our own detriment. As my friend noticed, parents spend so much of their time caring for their children that they end up sacrificing their own health and well-being in the meantime. If a parent has diabetes and has to cut back on sugar and limit their carbohydrates, they could feel torn between putting their whole family on a similar meal plan or eating differently themselves. I used to practice pediatric gastroenterology and took care of children with gluten allergies (celiac disease). Parents, stepparents, and other adults caring for children all told me, "It's just easier if the whole family follows a gluten-free diet." Navigating a change alone in a family can be difficult, whether you are the adult or the child, but sometimes you have to do that; maybe you have to take a special supplement or a medication or have to avoid a specific food because of an allergy. What you are doing for yourself, as a caregiver, may not be the right thing for your child. Parents who have shared their bariatric surgery story, including how they now have to eat small, protein-heavy meals, have come to realize that their meals will look different from the ones they may serve their children. It can lead to confusion and sometimes loneliness as they feed their family one meal and end up eating a different meal before or after the family. When it comes to our health, if we must follow a special diet, engage in specific exercises, or take a medication or supplement, we have to be careful when communicating these changes and figuring out the best way to navigate them within the household. Our children may not understand why we are doing these things, may be frightened by the health concern, or may try to copy behaviors without understanding why. This leaves us as parents with a quandary: Do we explain everything going on with our health, do we hide it, or do we settle somewhere in between?

Talking About Your Health (Not Weight) With Your Children

The principles for talking about bodies are similar to those for talking about your own health. If you are dealing with any health issues that require changing your health habits, here are a few tips in approaching the conversation with your children.

- **Be honest.** Explain the issues at hand and what changes you plan to make to address them. Continue to be careful about how you talk about food and health (particularly with younger children) to remove judgment about their eating or prevent fear of future problems. Instead of saying, "Daddy has high blood sugar levels because he used to drink a lot of sodas," explain what diabetes is and why Daddy has to eat less sugar *now*. If talking about high blood pressure, explain that a lot of things can cause high blood pressure (eg, genetic makeup, diet, stress), taking care not to blame yourself or something you used to do, like "I used to eat a lot of bacon and didn't exercise, so that caused me to get high blood pressure," thus avoiding equating a 1:1 relationship between a health habit and your blood pressure. This can scare children, which can either lead to overcompensation (your child avoids all sugar and displays signs of an eating disorder) or elicit the opposite reaction (eating a lot of sugar because they are scared it will be taken away from them). Finally, note that some efforts are just for adults and not necessarily for children: "Daddy's back sometimes hurts, so he is doing this special exercise to help manage that."
- **Keep things positive and within reason.** While we always want health changes to be for the whole family, every family is different. In our home, we go to work and school at different times, so we aren't able to have breakfast together on most weekdays. Our breakfasts differ because some of us prepare breakfast the night before to save time and the rest of us do it

that morning. If you change to a high-fiber breakfast to help with cholesterol, it's OK to say, "This food gives me energy—it's part of a balanced breakfast—and I like it. It will also help with my cholesterol." Or if switching up a workout routine, try "I do this exercise to be strong and help my body stay that way" or "Taking a walk helps me have a better day and not be grumpy after work." It's also not a requirement to provide reasons for a change. Some children, particularly younger ones, may not even ask why oatmeal is now being served a few days a week. A more common question is likely to be "Why can't we get breakfast from the drive-through on the way to school?" Your response can be as simple as "I'd like to have breakfast at home more often," without an in-depth discussion of cholesterol.

- **Talk about your own body as it is, without criticism or comparison to others.** For example, "I have a birthmark on my cheek. Sometimes I wish it wasn't there, but it's also a normal part of me, and I've grown to like it." When it comes to your health, keep body size and shape out of it. Criticizing our body or someone else's body implies that there are "good" and "bad" bodies. When you comment about someone else's weight gain or loss, the value of the weight change comes through to your children. Make sure your children hear you saying great things about your body even when you don't always love yourself. Having your child hear you say how much you love showing off your shoulders in a new dress conveys and teaches them self-confidence. Even better, express excitement about reaching a goal not related to your size: "I finally completed a 5-mile walk. I rock!"

- **Recognize and honor familial differences in bodies.** For instance, "My grandmother had the same hair as me. I love seeing her when I look in the mirror" or "Our family members all have a gap in their front teeth. Some have had braces to change the look. When I see my tooth gap, it reminds me of my father's smile!" For myself, my right eyebrow has these wild few hairs that grow straight up and curl, just like my father's. People comment on them and sometimes ask why I don't pluck or trim them; one person even reached up and tried to pluck them (*not cool!*). It would be reasonable and easy for me to trim those few eyebrow hairs, but I don't because they remind me of my father. Children may have inherited something about their bodies that they don't like and often can't change. Practicing loving their bodies, and not commenting negatively about them, can help them build up their own self-esteem and positive body image and learn to appreciate the uniqueness in everyone.

> **"I'm trying to lose weight. Do I explain this to my children?"**
>
> Whatever the reason is that you are trying to lose weight, it's important to know how to convey this to your children. Being a caregiver can sometimes make it more difficult to implement a change, so being aware of family dynamics can help you. Some studies show that young adults who developed disordered eating or a negative body image reported learning it in their own home, seeing the behavior start with their own parents. Knowing that eyes and ears are always watching and listening can help prevent any potential negative ripple effects on your children. I find it is helpful to share your reasons with children when you determine they have the maturity to understand. And it is important to link the weight loss goal to health or function, not to appearance or shame about size.

Discuss What Has Happened Since You Made a Change

Taking care not to equate a habit change 1:1 with a health improvement (because there won't always be a quick result), it's fine for you to note an improvement in making a change without focusing on weight:

Chapter 4 | Talking With Children About *Your* Health Changes

- "My blood pressure is starting to come down since I started walking in the mornings."
- "I am taking a lower dose of my cholesterol medication since we switched to ground turkey."
- "I think I'm less grumpy since I've started going to the gym at lunchtime."

"Should I talk with my children about my decision to lose weight?"

If you're going through bariatric surgery, participating in a weight loss program, or taking a medication that results in weight loss, there will likely be changes going on in your body and daily life that your children notice. These can be confusing for children and sometimes lead to worry or fear. If your body or habits or some other aspect of your daily schedule changes to the extent your child notices, it's better to address the situation before any concerns can develop by discussing the medical reasons for the change. Be honest about it, but don't feel obligated to make sure they understand all of it or have them be 100% correct in the physiology of your health condition. If the reasons or details are too personal, it's OK to be vague about it or come up with another way to explain it. After all, children share things with others we wish they wouldn't. Try to avoid telling them something that is not true. Listen to your own intuition and desire for privacy with what you share while still keeping in mind what your children are seeing and thinking. When having the conversation, keep it primarily focused on health:

- "I want to stay healthy, and this makes me stronger."
- "This new eating schedule keeps me energized all day."
- "I'm exercising often, so I need more water."
- "I've switched to cauliflower rice because of a doctor's advice. It is a tasty, easy switch to make, and it helps with my diabetes."

People's weight and health are very complicated, and it often takes several changes and time to see a difference. Some people cut out sugar-sweetened drinks (eg, sodas, juice, sports drinks), which is a great change to make, but it may not result in substantial weight loss. By focusing not solely on weight but rather on health, it sends a message to your children: "I made this change to better my health!"

Model the Behavior You Want to See in Your Child

Remember that modeling behavior is a very powerful way to influence the habits of your child. This fortunately will have positive ripple effects for your family, as you may prepare more meals at home, change the foods you buy at the grocery store, and add exercise to your routine. Regardless of your specific health journey, think about what habits are important to model for your children, such as eating regular meals at the table without distractions, drinking water, and scheduling time for exercise. Remember that you don't necessarily have to push or encourage these, but let the routine for your family develop naturally. Simultaneously, consider the things you may be doing that are not appropriate for your children to participate in: measuring portion sizes, counting calories, or frequently weighing yourself. In particular, continue to be alert about body and weight talk, which understandably may occur a lot when participating in a weight management program.

Some Habit Changes Are for the Family and Others Are Just for You

Just as alcohol is meant only for adults to drink, and your child's medications are meant only for them to take, there are habits that may be meant only for adults to have. Maybe you are drinking a protein shake as a meal substitute. While we don't recommend meal substitutions for young children, you can share that your shake is providing the nutrition your doctor recommended. For physical activity, this concept is quite pertinent. While many adults like walking on a treadmill (they can watch a TV show or avoid inclement weather), it would not come as a surprise that most children do not enjoy that. Luckily, there are plenty of age-appropriate options for children, such as sports and good old-fashioned outdoor play. If children are not involved with sports, there is a tendency to push adult-style exercise, such as exercise classes, treadmills, or stationary bikes. If your child wants to walk or run on the treadmill, that is great (for me, it's a great opportunity to catch up on movies while getting in some movement), but it's absolutely OK for them to *not* want to engage in this type of exercise. They are children and are not at a maturity level to recognize what to do to improve their health.

For some nutrition changes, these changes can be perfectly safe for children. For example, if you are trying to lower your cholesterol levels by switching from ground beef to ground turkey, it's perfectly fine to make that change for your family. There is no harm to your child to have less saturated fat in switching from beef to turkey. Most of the time, your family won't even notice the switch unless you mention it, so not mentioning it saves the hassle of you having to fix 2 different meals. If you are following a special diet, such as having a liquid, high-protein shake for a meal, share the reason with your family, as you feel comfortable, but do your best to still have the shake at mealtime with your family.

Weight Loss Medications

This is a newer situation, and there isn't a lot of research to go on, but we are listening to experts and the lived experiences from parents to share guidance with you. As we discussed in the "I'm trying to lose weight. Do I explain this to my children?" and "Should I talk with my children about my decision to lose weight?" questions earlier in this chapter, be honest and share what you are doing in age-appropriate language. Use your best judgment regarding their maturity to decide how much you discuss your weight loss medications with your child. You are entitled to privacy, so you do not have to reveal it all. Explain how the medication has been given for your health and will keep you healthy. Make sure to safely store all medication to prevent children from accessing it, and emphasize that this medication is *just for you,* and medications are not safe to share: "I'm using this medicine because it will help my body be healthy. My blood pressure and blood sugar levels are high, which can cause other problems, so I'm using this to help my body stay well and keep up with you!"

For older children who may have more questions, you can have a more detailed discussion about the matter. If your teen expresses interest in a weight loss medication for themselves, a visit to their doctor can be scheduled to discuss if that medication will be of help to them.

Linking the medicine to appearance only feeds into the idea that a lower weight or smaller body is the "acceptable" or "preferred" body and that you don't like your own body. Instead, explain how medicine helps your health in different, indirect ways, such as lowering blood pressure in order to prevent potential heart problems. In this case, medications for weight can help someone lose excess body fat, which can improve blood pressure. The goal of weight loss medication is to improve health over the long term. If your children notice you eat less at meals because of the medication, let them know you aren't as hungry and feel full. Guard against the instinct to use your decreased appetite as a way to set an example of how to eat less. For instance, avoid saying, "I'm listening to my body and trying to be healthy by not eating as much." Your child could interpret this comment as encouraging restriction, adding guilt to their appetite. Your children still need to eat the amount that is right for them. Continue to provide regular meals and snacks and eat together at the table as much as possible.

Bariatric Surgery

This procedure is similar to taking medications and changing habits to improve health. It's a step you are taking, as a parent, to improve your health. For most families, this will be an adults-only change, needed to help manage diabetes, improve mobility, and feel better. This may require you to do things a little differently than the family. Aside from talking about your surgery with your children, try to work together on the changes it may have in your role in the family. Eat meals together as a family, don't hide the nutritional changes associated with surgery, and turn to family for their support. At a minimum, sit with your child and family during the meal even if you are not eating or need to eat a special diet. The decision on how much to share about your surgery depends on either the age of your child and their ability to understand it or how private you want to keep it. In general, children younger than 7 years may have a harder time understanding the surgery and may not notice your lifestyle changes as much, so you may choose not to discuss it with them. You could use generalities: "Daddy has to have a surgery and will be home in a few days." Children aged 8 to 12 years may notice the surgery more, and you may choose to share more of what it is and why you are having it done, including what to expect after. Greater details can be shared with teenagers who have the capability of understanding the surgery and how it works. Generally, though, what is shared is up to you, so be as honest as you can and focus on how you can normalize the family routine to model healthy and safe behaviors.

Changing the Family Structure for the Better

The family unit, the family system, the family core, the family tree—there are dozens of ways we can describe how families are intertwined and linked together. And we don't mean just blood relatives; all families are unique and we all get to define who is in our family. A family living in the same home is inextricably linked to each other, so a change in one person will undoubtedly cause a change in another. Unfortunately for caregivers, family members can often interfere with those changes, not deliberately but naturally—just because of the complexities and uniqueness of families. Enlisting the support of the family can also help. Being open and honest about why you are making a change for yourself, or your family, takes away any confusion of why you are doing it. But like with Manuel in Chapter 3, (Not) Talking With Your Kids About Their Weight, discuss the changes matter-of-factly, such as in the following ways:

- "I need your help as I try to change some daily habits that will be hard for me. I'm going to start drinking diet soda and water instead of regular soda. My doctor says this will help me with my health."
- "I've been skipping breakfast because I'm tired in the mornings and need more sleep. I'm going to work on going to bed sooner so I can wake up in time for breakfast. I've learned this will help me eat enough throughout the day and have more energy. Getting more sleep and eating on a schedule are both hard for me, so I'm going to try hard to take care of my body in these ways."

- "I'm going to try taking a short walk after dinner. If you want to go with me, we can walk together sometimes. I want to exercise more, and walking after dinner is a great way to do it, but I need help to get into that habit, and I always love spending time with you."
- "I am going to be cooking more meals at home than I usually do. It will take some time for me to adjust to planning meals and buying groceries instead of ordering takeout. I'm looking forward to the change. I'm going to need a little patience from you all as I find what meals I can prepare that we all like." (Notice there is no mention of *healthy* in relation to food).
- "We're a team. When one of us needs help, we all chip in and work together. I need your help cooking dinner this Thursday."

It can be frustrating when we receive pushback while trying to do something beneficial for our families, like having more family meals. Be careful not to show that frustration.

"I work all day, then come home and cook, and all you do is complain about it!" is a phrase I've actually said to my children before—I'll admit it! Pushback is normal when making a change. Sometimes we can make a change without having to announce it, but sometimes it can help, particularly with older, more mature children, to bring them into the decision-making, so they are aware, and even task them with responsibility. It can end up making your job easier by spreading around the responsibilities (even something as simple as turning the oven on for you so it's preheated) so they can support what you are trying to do.

Be careful not to turn changes against them. For instance, avoid saying, "I want to eat better, but you only want to eat fatty food," as that will just lead to arguments and hurt feelings. This is where keeping a special meal (Spaghetti Night!) or event (Pizza and Movie Night!) in place can help ease these changes into place and convey the message about making small changes and not abandoning the more enjoyable activities around food.

Breaking the Generational Myths

Our children are watching us all the time, especially when we think they aren't. It's always amazing to me that I can yell for my sons to come to dinner and they never hear me, but the minute I whisper to my wife about something sensitive or private, suddenly they have the heightened hearing of a nocturnal fruit bat! Most of the time, though, they are learning all our positive qualities. But none of us are perfect; sometimes they pick up our less ideal habits too. Some of us grew up in times where it was OK to talk about someone's body or idealize the perfect figure. In more recent times, marketing companies are taking steps to show many different types of bodies and beauty, getting away from an idealized version that is unrealistic. Numerous studies have shown the harm that can occur, particularly in younger teens, in trying to achieve a certain appearance or body type.

Our children have the best chance of growing up without body shame when we support their bodies just as they are. Parenting in this way means changing the myths many of us were raised believing:

- Smaller bodies are better, prettier, and more accepted.
- People in larger bodies are lazy, unattractive, and less intelligent and eat too much—they did this to themselves!
- If we were smaller, we would be happier and healthier.
- Dieting and exercising are the best ways to change a larger body.
- Eating less takes willpower and self-control.
- We can lose weight if we try hard enough.
- If we are dieting and not losing weight, we must be cheating or lying about what we eat.

The first way to get rid of or prevent these myths from reaching your children is to model the new behavior yourself. Talk with the other adults in your family about following a new path to raising children, so family members don't make comments about bodies or share inaccurate health beliefs about supplements or a magic fat-burning exercise (Use this book in your argument!). Quietly and lovingly tell others we don't make comments about people's bodies, weight does not equal health, and we do things because we want to feel good and strong, not to weigh less on a scale.

What happened with Beverly and Jordan? Beverly and Jordan read an article about changing their relationship with their bodies. The article talked about how having more confidence with your body—as it already is—will make you happier and healthier. It also talked about not making comments about anyone else's body, because you don't know how those comments will be received. The two of them had some very intense, but helpful, talks between them. They decided to stop making comments about their bodies unless these were positive.

By changing how they talked about their bodies, Beverly and Jordan both saw improvements in how they felt about their bodies. They realized it took time to change the inner beliefs they had developed about themselves. Beverly began practicing making positive comments about her own body. She avoided comments about others who lost or gained weight. She praised Jordan for expressing themself with their unique clothes, showing off how confident they felt in a new outfit, or adding some fun to their look with colorful earrings. Comments now focused on how Jordan felt in a new look, not about how Jordan's body looked. Jordan no longer had to comment about how their mom looked in new clothes. The two of them still had to adjust and had some days of feeling more confident and other days of feeling dissatisfied with their bodies. It was a process, but the shifts had begun.

Chapter 5

Family Connection Is Your Greatest Strength

Teresa and Sheila have 2 children, Bryson and Lisa. Lisa is 12 years old, loves playing soccer, and likes to cook, just like one of her mothers. Bryson is 8 years old, is also an avid soccer player, and has very picky eating. Every meal is a struggle and usually results in him getting a granola bar and yogurt several times a day, as his parents think he has gotten too thin (although his doctor isn't worried). Mac and cheese is served with dinner almost every night, as that is one of the few things he eats that his parents cook.

During her yearly checkup, Lisa's doctor mentions that her weight is increasing a little too fast. The pediatrician says not to stress too much about it except limit the number of servings Lisa has of mac and cheese, serve smaller portions of the main meat entrée, and encourage more vegetables with dinner. Teresa is alarmed, as she has a history of weight struggles and doesn't want Lisa to have the same struggles, so she decides to follow the doctor's orders.

This makes Lisa feel very bad. She sees her brother snacking throughout the day, but when she asks for one snack, she is reminded of what the doctor recommended. Bryson can eat all the mac and cheese he wants, but Lisa is allowed only one serving. Lisa's other mother, Sheila, feels bad for Lisa. She cries to her often, so she takes her for milkshakes after soccer games and practices.

What are Teresa and Sheila thinking and feeling? This is hard! They have to balance getting Bryson to eat anything with trying to get Lisa on a healthier eating pattern. Dinners are already stressful because they are pushing Bryson to eat and upsetting Lisa, who can't have seconds. Sheila feels caught in between, wanting to help Bryson not be so picky and seeing how upset Lisa gets because they restrict her mac and cheese and portion sizes. She knows they are doing this to prevent Lisa from having problems with her weight later. Teresa remembers how she felt ashamed as a child for being larger than her sister, wishing she could fit into trendier clothes as a teen. In high school, she drank protein shakes to lose weight and remembers being hungry much of the time. She appreciates the medical advice to limit Lisa's eating so she won't grow up with a larger body, hoping it is the right answer for Lisa. Teresa is also worried that Sheila is not on the same page as her and is concerned they may be sending the children mixed messages.

What is Lisa thinking and feeling? Lisa is really upset! Bryson is picky and gets his favorite foods all day and mac and cheese every night, but Lisa is the one on the diet. Why is her weight a big deal but Bryson gets whatever he wants? What is she doing wrong? Why are her moms so mean about only one serving of mac and cheese? This is so unfair!

Things That Work Together

Parenting (be it biological parents, foster parents, stepparents, aunts, uncles, grandparents, or other caregivers) is key to your child's health and well-being. But other factors are at play than just your child and you as a caregiver: there may be another parent in the house, or other children, or there may be a grandparent or close friend helping out. Collectively, your child's well-being is most influenced by their family!

While we don't want to put you through a first-year Family Studies class in high school, one of the prevailing ways to understand families is as a system, or "things that work together," which I think is pretty accurate for a family. What is now generally referred to as *family systems theory* was developed in the 1960s by psychiatrist Murray Bowen, and in combination with other theories and research, to better understand and help families. There are many concepts to family systems theory that inform family-based treatments including family systems therapy, which continues to evolve over time. There are 3 components in particular that make it easier to understand why it can be difficult sometimes for families to make habit changes:

1. **Members of a family are connected.** While each person is unique, they are connected to other members of their family—brothers, sisters, parents, stepparents, foster and adoptive parents, and others. Sometimes those connections are tight, and other times they are loose, but there is always a connection. Within that family system, there are smaller systems. The family presented here is an example: Teresa, Sheila, Bryson, and Lisa are a family, all different ages, weights, and personalities. Bryson has a relationship with his sister, a different relationship with his mom, and a different one with his other mom. The same goes for the other members in his family. There are all these connections and relationships within the family; put them all together, and you have a whole family relationship. If Sheila wants to make a change in the family by cooking more meals at home, she needs to realize that it will affect everyone in the house, so she should take many things into account when making that change: What time does everyone get home so they can eat? Do they have time to cook because Lisa has soccer practice? Mom has an allergy to shrimp, so no recipe can contain shrimp. Will everyone like what Sheila is cooking? And so on. A simple change like cooking one more meal at home a week now has several more levels of complexity.
2. **Families interact with their environment and surroundings, and those surroundings affect us.** In short, families wanting to make changes will always be influenced by the world around

them. Sheila wanting to cook more meals at home and the family's work or school schedules both determine when they eat meals; she has to travel to a grocery store to get the ingredients, and if it isn't close, that will affect the plan. Sheila recently lost her job, so money is tighter and that influences what kind of foods they buy. Your family lives in the real world, and when making changes, you have to navigate that world as best you can.

3. **First- and second-order change.** This can be really complicated, but to break it down, there are 2 levels to change: first- and second-order. First-order change—of wanting to cook more meals at home—would be scheduling a night to cook dinner and pick out a recipe. That may not be hard to do once or twice, but turning that into a habit will take a second-order change, which can involve establishing the routine, cleaning off the dining room table for dinner, learning to cook more recipes, scheduling time to shop for ingredients every week and prepare the dinner, and carrying out a "no electronics at dinner" rule to talk and enjoy the meal. All of this takes more effort and will require more planning, conversations, and habit changes. Deeper changes to the family routine, rules, and communication patterns will be needed to make the changes stick.

Families are complicated and complex. Making changes as a family isn't easy, but understanding how families are connected will make it easier to make changes in the future. What is the magic ingredient? The secret sauce? The code? Simple: *communication.*

Communication within families is very, very important. Communication is more than just talking with each other. It's knowing what is going on in each other's lives. It's knowing how each other is feeling. It's talking in a way that the other person hears and understands you and choosing when it's actually an effective time to communicate. For example, my wife and I do much better planning for things (eg, meals, date nights, trips) in the morning when we are rested and not as rushed. If we try to talk at night, after a long day of work, we don't have the energy or concentration to plan anything, much less decide what we want to have for dinner. By the time we settle on dinner, we then have to see if we have the ingredients, make it, and serve it. By this time, it's late and we are getting ready for bed and preparing for the next day… which sometimes means "Fast food, here we come!"

Family communication is key but not easy. Household members are typically of different ages and will have different communication patterns. Especially in families that have moved to a new country, caregivers have cultural expectations, food and language that may differ from their children who have been raised in the new culture, and a different level of acculturation. Sometimes I do better at talking with my son by text; other times, in person; and still other times, just by listening to him (and not talking). Sometimes he isn't in the mood to talk, and if I force the issue, he shuts down. Some families communicate in different ways. No family will be the same, but it is vitally important to figure out how your family best communicates in order to make changes. It is normal for families to resist, or fight against, change (that is actually a part of family systems theory, that families do not naturally like change). Sometimes the best communication is knowing when and where to communicate; other times (eg, with teens), it's knowing when *not* to talk and just listen; and, for families that struggle with communication, it's simply starting the conversation.

The most important thing your family can do is to establish a schedule. As soon as you set a bedtime for your child, they will likely fight against it! Establishing a schedule (as detailed in Chapter 2, Parenting Through Structure and Love; see the "Does this apply to sleep too?" question) is really important for your children and you, and being able to effectively communicate is critical for your child to accept the schedule as a house rule.

Families Are Unique

There is no one definition of *family;* every family is different. Some might consider family only blood relatives, while others might consider close friends part of their family. My coauthors, Dara and Melissa, live near their parents and siblings, so they have a large extended family. I don't have family nearby, so we're a little different. About twice a

> week, we eat dinner with our close friends who live in the neighborhood, and our children were practically raised as brothers and sisters. So while we don't necessarily call them *family*, we see them more than most of our relatives and they have a big impact on our lives. Families don't have to be living in the same home, related by blood and genetic makeup, or structured as a traditional family. There are blended families, shared households, and multigenerational families. Family is whom you consider family; that is important because many nonrelatives will have an influence on you, your children, and your family. While you may not be able to change their personal habits, recognizing that they may influence your family's habits is important.

On the Same Team

A family is like a team, and often we play different positions on the team. In our own families, sometimes there are members in charge of dinner, those in charge of laundry, and so on. Like with any team, communication about jobs and tasks is key, including making sure caregivers know who is doing what and how they can support each other. One adult caregiver doing something different from the other can lead to problems; children may start going to one parent over the other when they need something. Clear communication between parents can allow them to support each other, be on the same team, and work toward the same goals for the family.

A common scenario we see is sabotage—when someone undermines what the other caregiver or adult in the home is doing, which is likely unintentional. When there are 2 or more adults involved and one adult does the opposite of what the other is doing, it is actually worse than doing nothing. This could be a sibling, a parent, a grandparent, another relative, or even a babysitter or family friend. These people usually don't purposely want to undermine the other, but it just ends up happening. It can be very confusing to children when 2 important adults in their lives are doing and saying different things. This is particularly important when households are blended or if children are living in 2 different households (eg, because of divorce, separation, or a need to split time between parents and grandparents). With different homes, families, and lifestyles, all caregivers really need to work together. Sometimes that isn't possible. If you co-parent with another person who lives in a separate home, different approaches to meal and sleep schedules, foods being served, and overall parenting are likely to occur. There have probably been discussions before in other areas of parenting, such as homework, bedtimes, and electronic use, and maybe mutual agreements at times were not reached, despite best efforts. Calmly explain to the other caregiver the changes you are making in your household, including why, and encourage their support in mirroring those changes in their home, as consistency will be best for your children. This may or may not occur in the other house, and in that case, continue to focus on what you can control, such as your routine and schedule. You can continue to communicate and focus on your household.

If conflict, disagreement, or different approaches to parenting around food, activity, and sleep is happening…then talk those out! Easier said than done, we know, but the sooner you get things in the open, the better. Take pressure off yourselves that you have to fix the disagreement in one night or one conversation. It can take time to work out new systems and change behaviors. It's about habits, and parenting involves habits as well. If you are like Sheila, sneaking out for milkshakes, don't cut off everything cold turkey, but work toward changing that by being open and discussing your concerns with your co-parent or co-parents. If you are the co-parent *not* going for milkshakes, don't come down hard on and shame your co-parent for doing that. Many caregivers aren't honest with each other because they expect this openness to lead to an argument or criticism. Some tips to get this started include

- **Set up a time to talk that will be focused on parenting;** you want to get on the same page as caregivers. Doing this when there isn't a lot of time to discuss the matter, or when another caregiver isn't expecting it, could lead to more tension or conflict.
- **Start out by saying that as parents, you are a team with the same goal:** it's about raising kind, caring, healthy children to be kind, caring, healthy adults. It's not about winning or getting your way but about doing what's best for your children.

- **Recognize that as a parent or caregiver, you will not always handle things in exactly the same way as a co-parent** (if there is one). Every team has different players and different positions. The running back can't play on the defensive line. Someone who swims the breaststroke probably won't swim the butterfly quite as well. Caregivers have different roles and positions to play, so even if you do something differently, you are on the same team and have the same goals: to be aligned, working together to raise great children, even if doing so in different ways.
- **Support each other:** come to an agreement to support each other, and make a promise not to undermine the other. Talk about parenting and developing the same approach, even if you differ slightly in how it is executed.
- **Don't criticize each other, either directly to each other or behind each other's backs**—and especially *not* to your children. Teams don't do well when they are criticizing each other and not working together.

Starting these conversations can be hard. If you aren't used to talking about being a parent, it can be uncomfortable. The same as for lifting weights: if you haven't lifted weights before, it's hard, it's uncomfortable, you don't feel very strong, and you will be very sore the next day. When you talk about your parenting approaches and raising children, it may feel awkward. But keep practicing it, and it will eventually become part of your family system. As we know, practice makes perfect: the more you do it, the better you will do.

The Relationship With Grandparents

For many families, grandparents are very important in the life of a family. In addition to passing down the family's history and traditions to grandchildren, they can be an immense help to parents, providing child care, emotional support, and unconditional love. They may also serve as primary caregivers when parents are unable to do so. In some families and cultures, grandparents serve a major role in raising and parenting as well. Multigenerational homes are common across the world and reflect the diversity and uniqueness of families. For the grandchild, there may be no people on earth more excited to see them than their grandparents. We all need that kind of love in our lives!

In our experience, parents love the support of grandparents and may question how their own stern parents became so lenient with their grandchildren! We hear often that a child's eating schedule and structure of eating at the table vanish when visiting grandparents. How do you handle this in partnership with grandparents? As with a co-parent, communication is a necessity.

If your child's grandparents live far away or see your child only a few times a year, keep those visits as special times, noting it's OK they bring your child that favorite cake or treat or take them to that favorite restaurant. In my culture, a grandparent's right is to spoil...and to build fun memories with their grandchildren! But they do need to respect your parenting rules, if the same is true in your culture. If you don't have sugary cereals at home and the grandparents are coming to visit or provide care for your children while you are traveling, let them know what you typically serve and then have it available.

If grandparents live close by and are very involved in your children's lives—for example, they provide babysitting, pick up grandchildren from school, and host regular sleepovers—communicate your routines so that grandparents can follow your house rules and schedule as best as possible. Allow them, however, to spoil the children periodically and offer the "dessert for breakfast" for your children. This can be a very tough conversation to have with grandparents; so, we recommend being gentle but clear and remaining flexible.

Making Changes as a Family

Making changes to our daily habits is hard enough, and doing it as a family system is even more complicated. The following points emphasize how to make the transition as smooth as possible:

- **Actions speak louder than words.** Communication is very important in families, but we also know that our children watch what we do. We must model for our children the behaviors we'd like to see. Studies show that our children will often adopt the habits we have. I often hear "I told my child to do that, but he won't listen." And when I say *often*, I mean that almost every day, I see patients and caregivers in my clinic who feel this way. Reminding children about a habit or change over and over doesn't work. A combination of setting expectations and modeling the behaviors you want to see will have a bigger impact.
- **Don't push too hard.** Remember the P & R Coin (see Chapter 2, Parenting Through Structure and Love, specifically the P & R Coin: Pressure and Restriction section)? When you push your family to make a change, you can receive pushback. Engaging in a power struggle with our children is frustrating. By removing the pressure and setting up structure for eating times, our children can make independent decisions about eating. There is a natural tendency as children grow to want predictability. They want to always have the same soft blanket on their bed or have a favorite glass for mealtime. As children have phases of wanting to work with you, engage them in changes like taking a walk together or learning a new recipe. These are also great ways to spend time with your children. It may feel like we have the most pushback from adolescents because they have growing verbal skills and quickly blossoming independence, especially when they can drive or use public transportation on their own. Even in these times, removing the pressure promotes more independent decision-making about eating.

- **Spend time together.** This is especially helpful for families that struggle to communicate. The best step to communicate more effectively is to spend more time together. Families can love each other very much and spend lots of time together but may not talk about things very openly. Every family is different, just like every basketball team in the NBA is different. There isn't a standard lineup, offense, or defense that makes a championship team each year; it's often not even the team with the league's best player. It's the team that plays the best together. The best athletes in the world will likely be beaten if they don't practice together! (Look up the 2004 USA Olympic basketball team: the best collection of basketball players in the world, heavily favored to win the gold medal, but who were beaten badly.) Plan time to be together, whether it is eating a meal, going to a movie, playing a board game, or completing household chores to your favorite music. Spending more time together will result in more communication between family members, and overall, things will work a little smoother. In our clinic, we usually start with board games or card games that everyone is familiar with. This approach leads to families spending dedicated time together and communicating more, which eventually makes implementing change easier.

Throughout the World

Most of the key research in families and weight, and our experience, is limited to North America. Weight, nutrition patterns, and physical activity vary throughout the world. As mentioned in Chapter 2, Parenting Through Structure and Love (see the A Scientific Approach to Parenting section), parenting approaches to child-rearing can be quite different between cultures and countries. Always take your family's history and traditions into account when making changes to improve health, as you don't want to lose or change the qualities that make your family who they are.

You Can't Spell "Teamwork" Without "Work"

Sometimes families might have trouble getting along or the family's personality differences can lead to more conflict; thus, more time together may make things worse. This can be especially true for siblings who argue. There are different approaches you can take as a caregiver to build cohesion if conflict arises in your family:

- **Find something everyone likes and do it together.** This is sometimes easier said than done, but if there are relationship challenges (eg, arguments, differing personalities), think about something fun that can neutralize the situation, such as going to the movies or watching a movie at home (although choosing which movies can be tough, so as a parent, you take the lead on that). While watching a movie doesn't encourage communication, it sets the foundation for spending time together.
- **Choose an activity without competition or teams.** If competition is building rivalry and hurt feelings, shift to noncompetitive options. Understand there will be pushback, eye-rolling, or grumpy comments, but stay positive and keep at it. In my family, we used to play board games, but sometimes that led to competition, arguments, or cheating accusations. We shifted to games that had us compete against ourselves and were fun. One board game involved making up definitions of words, and we had to guess who was telling the truth. It was silly and defused the competition between our children.
- **Spend one-on-one time with each child.** This can help establish communication and a stronger relationship. This is time to listen, and each child has their voice heard. Schedule dates or special activities when you are able. Give your child your undivided attention to communicate how important this time is and that you are paying attention without any distractions. Consider instituting a regular time each week or month that is "your night" with that family member.
- **Prioritize meals together.** Establishing regular family meals is a huge step toward the goal of spending time together. I can promise you, years from now, they will remember it positively.

- **Consider family therapy.** If conflict between family members can't be overcome, consider talking with a family therapist or mental health professional, who can help figure out why conflict keeps happening and provide more individualized guidance on how to improve the family dynamics. Seeing a counselor or therapist may be uncomfortable or new but can be incredibly helpful in the long run.
- **Control what you can control.** When conflict arises, make sure everyone is being heard and address ways to build cohesion.

> **What about Teresa, Sheila, Bryson, and Lisa?** Everyone is miserable! Teresa and Sheila are struggling with encouraging Bryson to try new foods, and Lisa seems sadder at every meal. The first step is to lift everyone's spirits. Teresa and Sheila decide to switch their approach. With guidance from a dietitian, they create a schedule for meals and snacks to support the picky eating behavior and the weight concerns. They also avoid discussing anything regarding food. Lisa isn't restricted, and they stop pushing Bryson to try new foods (mac and cheese is still on the table). This seems to improve many of their moods. Next, Teresa and Sheila set up rules around meals that everyone has to follow, such as *not* offering an "alternative dinner" that is fixed if someone doesn't like what is being served. Teresa and Sheila make sure that there are several things being served with each meal and there is something in the meal Bryson will eat, without them having to make an entirely separate meal just for him. In-between meal snacks are still not allowed unless the snack is their after-school one.
>
> Despite some initial pushback and frustrated talk (especially from Bryson, who is used to on-demand snacks all day), the children settle into this new routine. Their parents immediately notice less sneaking of food by Lisa, and the meals are a bit more peaceful. Slowly, Bryson starts trying

new foods when he realizes his yogurt and granola bars are limited to after school; he remains hungry just before dinner and understands there won't be more food until breakfast. Teresa and Sheila are now working as a team with their parenting around eating. Their messages are consistent and they both like the decreased tension at meals. It is a slow transition, but mealtimes improve significantly, and new habits are being developed.

CHAPTER 6

Small Shifts, Big Impact: Transforming How Your Family Eats

Liz is a busy mom of 3 boys, Tim, Chris, and Steve, aged 9, 11, and 14 years. Liz was just diagnosed with high blood pressure and was told to cut back on salt, eat more fruits and vegetables, and add more whole grains and lean proteins. That night, she announces to her sons "No more eating out; we are eating healthy at home!" The boys protest all the way through dinner, which hurts her feelings, and the meal ends in silence when they realize how upset she is.

While cleaning up, Liz thinks about how many times she has been told *what* to do by her doctor, friends, and magazines; she realizes that as the mom of 3 boys, no one has ever told her *how* to do it.

What is Liz thinking and feeling? Frustration, frustration, frustration! Some days she feels in a rut, while other days she feels powerless to make a change. She also worries about her sons growing up with "bad" eating habits and about how dinners at home aren't fun anymore.

What are the boys thinking and feeling? They are definitely annoyed! Why does their mom's new diagnosis have to mean they change everything? They enjoy being able to eat out. This means all their meals will be gross.

When it comes to eating, we like to focus on 3 simple habits: eat on a schedule, cook at home, and eat together. In this chapter, we'll talk about why these habits are important and share easy tips to help your family make changes—without losing the fun and joy of food.

Eat on a Schedule

Children and teens thrive on structure, and having a consistent eating schedule is just as important as maintaining a regular work or school routine.

Set a Schedule

If your family doesn't have a general schedule for meals and snacks, this is a great time to start. Allowing your children to transition to eating on a schedule is important in the following ways:

- **Reliable eating schedules help us come to meals hungry, but not too hungry.** When children come to meals hungry, they are more likely to eat the foods you've prepared and even try new foods. When children are overly hungry, it can cause them to eat too fast and even eat more than their body needs.
- **Children tend to do better with their eating when they know what time the next meal or snack will be served.** There is a level of comfort children feel when they know what to expect. Especially if there is any history of trauma or food insecurity, predictability in this way provides security.
- **Children become less obsessed with food, especially younger children, when meal schedules are in place.** If children aren't sure when their next meal or snack is, it can lead to them thinking about food too much and even lead to food preoccupation or thinking about food all the time. They may take every opportunity they can to eat and snack, even when they aren't hungry.
- **We learn to recognize our hunger when our body is on a meal schedule.** If your children eat regular meals and snacks, they begin to recognize feelings of hunger. Our bodies learn to eat, then wait, then eat, then wait throughout the day. On the

other hand, grazing promotes the opposite behavior. Grazing prevents opportunities for noticing hunger, and we gradually begin to lose a sense of when we are truly hungry. For some children, grazing or frequent snacking can ruin their appetite for their next meal, and for others, it can lead to overeating throughout the day. Eating on a schedule, even if it ends up being slightly modified to fit the schedule of the family, helps children develop typical hunger patterns. Given predictable times to eat, children adapt to the schedule and their bodies learn to eat enough at each meal or snack time to last until the next eating time.

> **A Simple Reminder: Model the Habits You Want to See**
>
> Modeling eating on the schedule is an important piece. When our children see us eating, they will also want to eat. And when they don't see us eating, they may learn that skipping meals is acceptable.

As children become older and schedules a little busier, you adjust and do the best you can in setting up times for people to eat. It's somewhat common for teenagers to skip breakfast as their sleep cycle starts to shift a little later and school regulates meal and snack times during the day. But set the expectation that there are set times to eat at home. Implementing the expectation that your family eats only during meal and snack times can set the foundation for your child to develop healthy habits.

Offer 3 Meals a Day at Set Times

If you are building this habit, don't stress too much about *what* you are serving at first; you are simply trying to establish the habit of eating meals at a set time.

- Set regular times for eating every 3 to 4 hours, including a snack between meals if there is more than a 4-hour gap.

- Mealtimes may vary depending on evening activities, so adjust the schedule as needed.
- Model eating on the schedule. Sit down and eat with your children.

A simple guideline is to offer 3 to 4 food groups at each meal (the balanced meal), including protein, a grain/starch, and fruit and/or a vegetable. This gives you the opportunity to introduce new foods: serve a familiar protein and vegetable, and experiment with a new recipe for a grain. Don't feel like you have to remove foods from your meals to fit traditional rules or expectations. Who says you can't have fruit for dinner and a vegetable with breakfast? I noticed a huge difference at our own dinner table when we started putting a bowl of grapes out during the evening meal and when my son started fixing peanut butter and jelly sandwiches for breakfast in high school.

Offer 1 to 2 Snacks at Set Times

For families with children in school, this refers to the after-school snack. Younger children may need an additional morning or evening snack. There is no magic to the time except recognizing that snacks serve to bridge long gaps between meals and keep us from becoming too hungry. Try to eat snacks at the same time each day. Avoid allowing children to graze on food at any time, even if it's fruit or another item considered healthy, as that will still interfere with their typical hunger-and-eating cycle. Instead, include the following foods at the set snack times:

- Include 2 food groups with each snack. This approach helps serve the overall purpose of a snack: to be a bridge between meals. Combine a cheese stick with an apple or crackers or mix yogurt with some granola. Use the food you have and what's affordable. This can be a tortilla with cheese or peanut butter that you spread on crackers.
- Save sweet options, like cookies and ice cream, for dessert.
- Your child can choose to skip the snack, but if they do, they'll need to wait until the next scheduled eating time.

Eat Only at Meal and Snack Times

Keeping to meal and snack times can be the most difficult to put into place. It's always hard to figure out if your children are feeling hungry or if they are responding to seeing a favorite food. My oldest son once saw us packing snacks for a Super Bowl party, and he immediately said, "I'm hungry; can I have some of that?" When we told him no, but he could have his regular after-school snack of cheese and crackers, he declined. He wasn't *actually* hungry; he just wanted the special Super Bowl snacks and thought saying he was hungry would result in us forking over the Super Bowl snacks. If your children eat on a regular schedule and allow themselves to get hungry between meals and snacks, it will reinforce the routine and help protect against grazing.

- Between eating times, water and sugar-free drinks may be offered.
- When age-appropriate, involve your children in setting the eating schedule. This increases their likelihood of following it. If reminders are needed, post the meal schedule where everyone can see it, and let the schedule guide the family.
- When children ask for food between eating times, help them by pointing them to the next eating time on the schedule.

What About Hunger Between Meals?

Beginning in the toddler years, favorite, indulgent, or highly palatable foods can lead to eating when not hungry, otherwise referred to as *eating in the absence of hunger*. Around 7 or 8 years of age, children are similar to adults in that external cues (eg, seeing, smelling, or thinking about food) can set off their hunger. Eating on a schedule also helps with frequent snacking. We know it can be a big struggle for caregivers (and we have observed it is especially hard for grandparents who help with caregiving) when they are trying to make changes in eating habits and children are saying they're hungry. It may seem like you are denying them food, but it teaches them regular eating patterns and routines. It also keeps them open to new foods by coming to meals hungry.

> ### Respect Your History With Food
>
> We recognize that denying food to your child can really tug at your heartstrings. It may be a reminder of past times when you experienced not eating enough. If you went to bed hungry as a child, it may cause great anxiety to send your own child to bed hungry just because the timing isn't right. Please respect your own history with food. This can create a deeper emotional response than you may expect from yourself. If feelings about denying food to your child are overwhelming, adjust the schedule. Provide an additional evening snack time in your schedule so that a child who is not eating at dinner still has another time to eat before going to sleep. The goal is to have a set schedule. It is OK for the caregiver to adapt the schedule when the times aren't working well.

A frequent situation we hear about is when children eat lunch early at school and come home famished. A little investigation on your end can help: Are they eating their entire lunch at school? What is the snack they receive? It may not be filling enough or bridging the long gaps between meals. In the end, after some investigation, it may help to offer a snack when they get home. Some families eat dinner in the late afternoon or early evening, right when their children arrive home from school, so as not to interfere with practices, part-time jobs, or other activities. In that case, an after-school snack may not make sense, but an evening snack, several hours after dinner, may be more appropriate. Families may adjust the eating schedule for religious observances, such as Ramadan, by fasting during the day and planning together for the iftar, the meal shared at sunset.

Cook at Home

To eat more meals at home, the first step is planning. That can look different for every family. Maybe you're great at planning but have trouble following through. Or maybe planning feels hard because of a busy schedule. You might already plan well but want new ideas to make the process easier. No matter where you are, we're here to help!

A Plan in Advance Is Key

So why is planning recommended when it can feel so overwhelming to do? The benefits, as outlined in the following list, make it worth it:

- **Save time.**
    - *Avoid the stress of last-minute cooking;* otherwise, cooking will usually take longer while you try to determine if you have everything you need.
    - *Take fewer grocery trips.* When you are ready to cook, everything is there. No last-minute run to the store.
    - *Thaw food ahead of time.* If you plan to make a fish or chicken dinner the following day, place it into the fridge the day before so it will be ready to use by the time you cook the following day.
    - *Task other family members to be part of the meal prep.* An oven takes a while to preheat, so having someone turn it on while you are driving home can save time in the evening. My oldest son arrived home before we did when he was in middle school. We would call and ask him to take things out of the refrigerator, preheat the oven, and even get water boiling for pasta.
- **Save money.**
    - *Stick to your grocery list to avoid impulse buys that may go bad or spoil before you have time to use them.* Studies show that if you don't have a prepared list, you are more likely to be influenced by ads.
    - *Shop sale items.* Checking out discounts online, through a store's app, or in the store flyer can result in saving a lot of money.
    - *Plan for leftovers.* Make double protein one night, then use some the next night in a different dish.
    - *Consider online grocery shopping.* Planning meals can help you place an online shopping order and stick to a certain

dollar amount at checkout. More grocery stores are offering this, and you will save a lot of time by picking the groceries up in a matter of minutes through options such as curbside pickup. Shopping online can also help avoid the temptation of adding extra items to your cart that may find their way there while you are at the store. But if you are like me, you don't have to fully shop online. I am very, very picky about my bananas and apples, so I buy those once a week at the store and then use online shopping for a second trip during the week for some fresh items to cook with that I'm not as particular about.

- **Add variety to meals.**
    - *Meals can include more than 1 to 2 foods.* A one-pot stew that has protein, vegetables, and rice is a well-rounded, balanced meal that is likely to give leftovers if you double the recipe. Even if there is a family member in the house who has picky eating, still move forward with the stew. By planning ahead, you can serve it with a salad, fresh fruit, and some toasted bread. This gives other options to them, without making a whole separate meal for them.
    - *Make one meal everyone can eat.* For busy families, it can be hard to find time to shop and cook a meal, much less make a separate meal for everyone. No one has time to be a short-order cook! Having a separate meal sets the expectation that you will keep doing so in the future and will only make picky eating even pickier. Discussing the meal plan ahead of time, creating a list of favorite meals, and offering a few items with every meal keep everyone on the same page and allow you to make only one meal a night.
    - *Include familiar foods with new foods.* It's natural for some children, and even adults, to be wary of new foods. One reason why some efforts to change family habits do not work is that we start cooking all kinds of new recipes, and the "newness" of them scares off some members in the family. A common tip that restaurant chefs give is to pair newer or unfamiliar foods with familiar foods. If you eat at a restaurant, try finding a protein or meat on the menu that sounds exciting

or is unfamiliar to you, and look at the side dishes because the protein is likely being served with very familiar side items. It might inspire you and any future dishes you make!

In our clinic, we encourage families to begin by focusing on *how* they are eating. This means establishing consistent eating routines and allowing their child to decide how much to eat. Once this foundation is in place and families feel ready, we can begin to shift attention to *what* they are eating. Families can advance to serving a variety of foods to create a balanced meal, making sure to offer a protein, a starch/grain, and fruits and vegetables so children have several foods to choose from during the meal (Figure 6.1). We understand that isn't always possible given the foods available to your family (may not have that many food groups in the home), the situation (traveling or living somewhere temporarily), or health considerations in your child and family (food allergies). We are certain that you are doing your best and encourage you to find the parts of this guidance that work best for you.

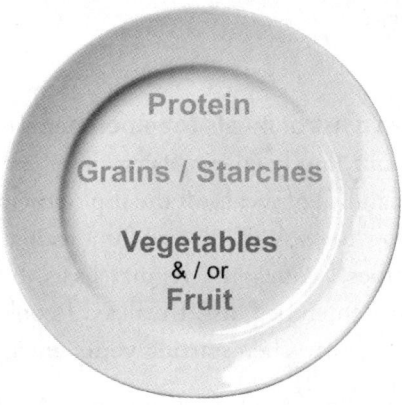

Figure 6.1. Balanced Meal

The At-Home Meal Playbook

There are many ways to plan meals. Below is one method families find to be especially effective for maintaining consistency over time and turning meal planning into a lasting habit.

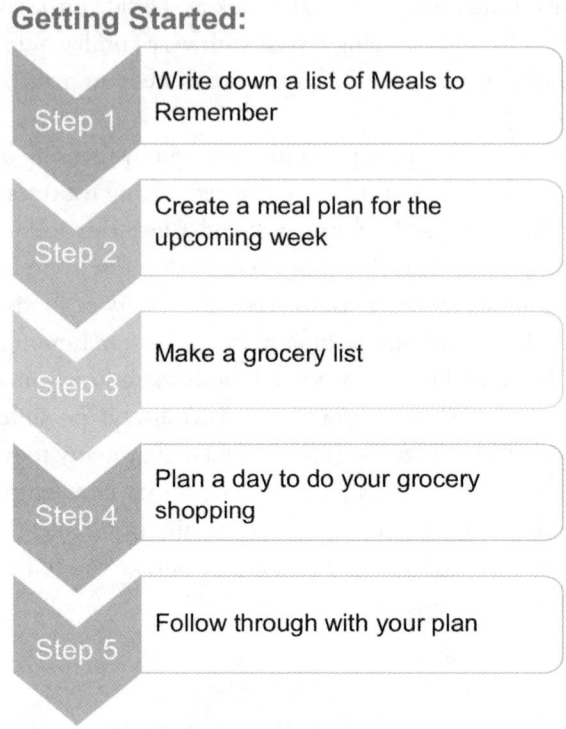

Step 1: Write down a list of meals to remember. This is a list of foods, recipes, or meals your family enjoys. Typically, the average person will remember only a handful of meals off the top of their head when asked, much less know how to cook them without a recipe. I can name about only 10 to 12 recipes I cook on a regular basis, but after looking at my own "Meals to Remember" list, I realized I cooked more than 100 different recipes last year! When starting yours, include

- A mix of healthful options, family favorites, and culturally familiar recipes that your family enjoys
- Foods that are affordable and easy to find at grocery stores
- Foods that are easy to prepare and fit into your schedule

Figure 6.2 provides an example of how you might write out your list. Your food list will likely differ, as the example does not encompass the full range of cultural food practices and traditions.

Chapter 6 | Small Shifts, Big Impact: Transforming How Your Family Eats

Meals to Remember

Entrées
Spaghetti
Teriyaki chicken
Tacos
Chicken soup
Homemade pizza
Chicken curry
Lentils
_____
_____

Sides
Rice
Mac and cheese
Roasted vegetables
Fruit salad
Green beans
Broccoli
_____
_____

Figure 6.2. Example of a "Meals to Remember" List

If you're looking to incorporate new recipes, go for it! We, however, recommend limiting these recipes to no more than one per week. New recipes often take extra time and effort to prepare, which can make it harder to stick to your plan if something unexpected disrupts your schedule.

Tip From Joey

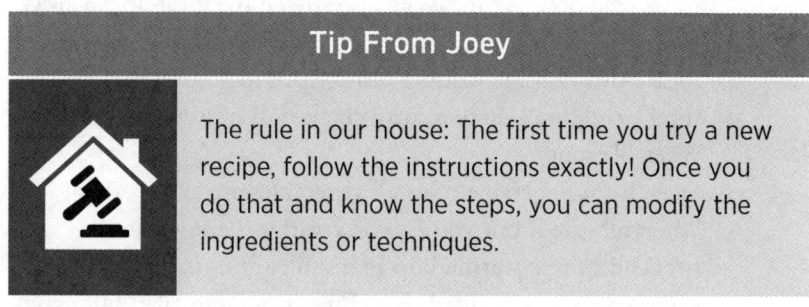

The rule in our house: The first time you try a new recipe, follow the instructions exactly! Once you do that and know the steps, you can modify the ingredients or techniques.

Step 2: Create a meal plan for the upcoming week. Depending on your needs, this may be a plan for the full week or just a few days at a time. Here are important steps to consider in your planning...and don't forget to use the family system (explained in Chapter 4, Talking With Children About *Your* Health Changes; see the Changing the Family Structure for the Better section)!

- **Have leftovers.** Decide which night(s) will be dedicated to leftovers (people call these "planned-overs"). This can also be a "clean out the fridge" night, where everyone eats a different leftover from earlier in the week. (We call that Smorgasbord Night).
- **Cook simple meals.** Have a few go-to quick meal ideas on hand for busier nights. Maybe you opt for grilled cheese with tomato soup and some fruit on the side. Ready in 15 minutes!
- **Decide who cooks.** Recruit some help from family members. It does not have to be you executing every meal. Children or other adults in the home can start the meal, do some prep before you get home, or even just start heating up some of the leftovers.
- **Maximize your budget.** Repurpose ingredients for future meals and consider swapping out certain items for more affordable alternatives.
  - Stretch the protein. Plan for one meat or protein to last multiple meals. Start with a "big" meat, such as slow-cooked pot roast for your first meal, and use leftover meat to make 3 more meals for the week. Using plant-based proteins for those who don't eat meat can also stretch the meal. Inexpensive proteins such as tofu or beans can add extra servings to your meal. Also, consider adding black beans to ground beef taco meat or adding tofu to a curry chicken dish. Add quinoa to vegetable soup.
  - Stretch the vegetable. Not all vegetables are as appetizing when reheated, but you can be creative. Oven-roasted broccoli can be warmed up in a skillet and made crispy or even have a sauce added to it. Prepare a large salad but avoid adding dressing to the entire bowl to prevent sogginess. Instead, have everyone add theirs individually. Seal it tightly and have it for tomorrow's lunch or as the vegetable at dinner the following night.
  - Stretch the grain/starch. Roasted potatoes are a favorite in my house, so we always make double. The next night, you can chop them finer and make a potato salad with a simple

salad dressing or you may have leftover rice that works well for hibachi fried rice. Leftover corn-on-the-cob can also be repurposed. Cut the kernels off the cob; add a little chopped onion, a can of diced tomatoes, and a cup of lima beans; and cook in a little oil to create a southern vegetable dish called *succotash*. Or heat a little oil in a pan and crisp the corn kernels.

- **Pick a theme night.** Simplify your planning by picking theme nights, like Taco Tuesdays. This helps narrow down options and adds fun to the meal. Figure 6.3 is an example of a weekly meal plan. This is not a prescribed diet plan for your family but a template on how theme night could look for your family.

Meal Theme Nights

Sunday: Slow Cooker	Monday: Meatless Monday	Tuesday: Mexican	Wednesday: Noodle Night	Thursday: Snacks and Game Night	Friday: Pizza	Saturday: Off-the-Grill
Chicken chili	Chipotle black bean burrito bowls	Tacos	Thai chicken with peanut noodles	Chicken nachos	Homemade flatbread pizza	Burgers and grilled vegetables
French dip sandwiches	Veggie stir-fry with tofu	Enchiladas	Spaghetti with meatballs	Veggies and dip Chips and salsa Fruit and dip	Order pizza	BBQ pork chops

Figure 6.3. Meal Theme Nights Example

- ○ Get takeout. When you do choose a day for going out, consider bringing home the meal and having it at the table just as you would when you cook at home.
- **Stock your fridge or freezer.** Stock up on sale items like meat, frozen vegetables and fruit, or bread. Choose a day to prepare a freezer-friendly meal, or prep meals in advance that can be frozen and easily reheated when needed.
  - ○ Roasts can be kept in the freezer for up to 12 months before being used. That's 3 times as long as ground beef!

> ### Fun Fact
>  Frozen veggies are picked at peak ripeness and retain their vitamins and minerals longer.

Step 3: Make a grocery list. Make sure to review what you already have in your home. My wife came up with the term "guess-shopping" to refer to when you shop without checking what you already have. You put ketchup on the grocery list because it's a key part of the BBQ chicken recipe for Tuesday night. You pick up a bottle at the store, check it off your list, and come home only to realize you already had 2 bottles—guess-shopping!

Step 4: Plan a day and time to do your grocery shopping. As you begin cooking more regularly, having the ingredients you need on hand is essential. Picking up items daily can be time consuming, and many of us don't schedule dedicated time to shop. Choosing a consistent shopping day (or two) each week can help you stick to your routine. Online grocery shopping can be a great tool for meal planning, although some people prefer selecting items in person (I'm obsessed with finding just-the-right banana!). That said, shopping habits vary widely. For some, weekly shopping isn't realistic—especially when transportation is limited. In those cases, you may do a large shopping trip every 2 to 4 weeks and make smaller trips for essentials like milk, bread, and produce. On the other hand, if kitchen storage space is limited, more frequent shopping is often necessary. The key is to find a rhythm that works for your household and supports your meal planning goals.

Step 5: Follow through with your plan. This follow-through usually starts with the grocery shopping, but for some not used to cooking often, there may be some stop-and-go with this habit. Stick with it as best as possible. It's OK to shift a meal or two around for the week because you already have all the groceries at home. Give yourself some grace. Build time into your schedule to prepare food.

Chapter 6 | Small Shifts, Big Impact: Transforming How Your Family Eats

"I'm not a good planner. How can I change this?"

Our lives don't always fit into nice and tidy schedules—some of us work weekends, others work evenings or overnight, and some schedules change all the time. You aren't a bad parent if you don't have the entire month planned out ahead of time; that is OK.

Tip 1: Start small.
If you're struggling to plan meals for the week, begin with one meal like breakfast. Put a to-do list on your refrigerator: "At the grocery store, buy bananas and yogurt for breakfast." Plan just 1 to 2 dinner meal days for the week to start. You can build from there. Add quick dinner options that are easy to prepare and offer flexibility when your schedule shifts, such as spaghetti and frozen green beans (pantry/freezer staples) or quesadillas with rotisserie chicken and salad.

Tip 2: Be flexible.
If Wednesday's dinner plan falls through, try it again on Thursday.

Planning isn't about perfection—it's about having options.

Tip 3: Have grace.
It's not a failure if you don't make or follow the plan each week. Start fresh the next day or next week. The path to change doesn't mean keeping the train on the tracks the entire time. It's expected for the train to be off track at times. Getting back on track is what builds real habits. The planning part is all about focusing on having more meals at home. Being prepared and having a game plan, even if you don't have a schedule in place yet, will do wonders to assist with this transition. "Out of sight, out of mind" is a big part of cooking at home. If you aren't sure about what is planned

for dinner, you are much more likely to buy food from the drive-through. If your children push back against some of your changes by begging to get takeout often, you can refer to the meal plan. Children are much less likely to push back if they know the rules and know there is a schedule for the week (ie, if they know what to expect), such as seeing that Thursday night is Takeout Night. Also, if things are posted or lists are made, there is a constant reminder. Having things posted makes them easy to remember. If you don't have a calendar of meals for the week (Figure 6.4), you can still take important steps to help make cooking more prominent in your home, such as the posted grocery list or the "Meals to Remember" list.

Weekly Family Meal Plan

Sunday	Monday	Tuesday	Wednesday	Thursday	Friday	Saturday
Chicken alfredo (Use leftover chicken) Salad Grapes	Frozen pizza Raw broccoli and carrots Vegetable dip	Beef and broccoli stir-fry Rice Pineapple	Leftovers	Turkey sloppy joes Sautéed asparagus Strawberries	Out to eat	Chicken with beans and rice Tortillas Lettuce, cucumbers, and tomato Mango

Evening Activities

	Scouts		Soccer		Soccer	

Who's Cooking?

Parent	Teen	Parent		Parent		Parent

Figure 6.4. Weekly Family Meal Plan

Chapter 6 | Small Shifts, Big Impact: Transforming How Your Family Eats

> **"I don't like to cook. What can I do?"**
>
> We get it. Some people do not like to cook. While we would encourage anyone to have a few dishes up their sleeve, we understand that for some families, this may not be possible. In the long run, it will still be better and cheaper to *prepare* and eat more meals at home. And you can still raise your children to like a variety of foods, even if you don't cook a lot, but you can achieve the goal of eating more meals at home. Frequently eating out in restaurants or drive-through establishments presents the challenge of your children always ordering the same items, thus not being exposed to a lot of different foods. This can cause a problem if they eat dinner at a friend's house or when they leave your house and are on their own: they won't be able to make do with other potentially unfamiliar foods.

If you really don't enjoy cooking, there are still some things you can do to eat meals together as a family at home, as much as possible. The following steps, or phases, will make the transition easier:

- **Phase 1: Eat at home.** Pick up already-prepared food, such as from the deli section of the grocery store, and bring it home so you can eat together at the table. This sets the foundation for the family eating the same meal, as well as the building blocks toward creating the family mealtime routine. Even when enjoying takeout, bring it home to have it with the family!
- **Phase 2: Prepare or assemble a meal at home.** Notice we didn't say *cook*. Cooking is great, and we want more people to cook meals at home, but if you don't have the time, or haven't learned the skills yet, assemble the meal and place it onto the table. This could be an already-cooked rotisserie chicken and a salad kit or "bagged salad," where everything is already cut and comes with a packet of salad dressing. It may be a frozen lasagna that can go straight from the freezer into the oven (and

may even have enough for another night of leftovers). This is one step closer to enjoying home-cooked meals than eating at a restaurant, and it can save you a lot of time. It also doesn't have to be fancy or complicated, maybe sandwiches and canned fruit. The goal is to have a meal, partially or mostly prepared or assembled at home, on the table for your family. This is preferred to takeout or restaurant meals, and you're still eating together at home!

- **Phase 3: Cook one part of the meal.** Once you have navigated the first 2 phases, try cooking one part of the recipe or meal. You can always include an assembled meal, like chicken and an already prepared salad. The most cost-effective and healthful thing to do, however, is to cook, prepare, or assemble more of your own meals. For some of us, we didn't take a home economics or cooking class; maybe our caregivers or grandparents may not have shown us how to cook; or we simply don't like cooking. All of that is understandable, so don't get down on yourself about it. The goal is to spend more time together as a family over a meal. If you are interested in trying to cook more, there are thousands of videos and recipes in books or online that provide cooking instructions whether you are the novice cook or an experienced chef. If you are new to cooking, we recommend opting for simple recipes with less than 10 ingredients and 10 steps, and there are plenty of tasty recipes out there with fewer than 5 of each.

Joey's Favorite Weeknight Salad

We like to share the following simple salad recipe, which pairs well with any meat or protein, especially if you like to grill:

- Lettuce/arugula—about 5 ounces. You can buy it prewashed in a bag or plastic container.
- Olive oil—3 tablespoons, or 3 one-second pours.
- Balsamic vinegar—2 teaspoons, or 1 one-second pour.

> - Minced garlic—either 1 clove of garlic chopped up fine or 1 teaspoon of minced garlic from a jar.
> - Salt and pepper—to taste, or start with about ½ teaspoon of each, then add more later if you like.
>
> Mix the olive oil, vinegar, garlic, and salt and pepper together in a large bowl; add the lettuce or arugula (or a mix!); and toss with a pair of tongs. Taste to see if the salad needs anything else, and serve it with any of your favorite meats on top and grains on the side.

Cook One Meal for All

We can oftentimes find ourselves in the habit of preparing multiple meals for different family members. This may start because we are catering to a family member with picky eating, feeding an infant or a toddler, or feeding someone with specific food preferences. When we do this, our children are exposed less to new foods, and over time, there will be fewer and fewer foods they will eat. If children are used to having the same few foods, over and over, it makes it even harder to try a new dish. This results in us coaxing, begging, tricking, and even trying to force them to try a new food. All of this backfires, we promise you—any of those things can lead to children liking the food even less. So what do we do? We don't want our children to have picky eating, and parents end up being what is commonly called a "short-order cook," making different dishes for every member of the family. Also, in our experience, when everyone is eating different dishes for meals, they start to not eat together, as Dad will cook one dish for the oldest child, who will start eating, while the younger child is waiting for Dad to finish the second dish—and so on.

If your family is used to cooking different dishes for different people every night, it can be difficult to change. The following list offers tips on breaking out of that habit:

- **Start slowly.** Have one meal per week where everyone eats the same meal.

- **Have a Leftover Night.** If you cook 2 to 3 times a week, there will likely be several dishes available for this theme night. Family members can choose from several leftover foods.
- **Include 1 to 2 foods at the meals that you know your child likes and can fill up with.** It is OK for them to skip some items. For example, if dinner is baked chicken, mac and cheese, green beans, strawberries, and milk, don't get too caught up in them tasting or eating everything on the table. Remember, pressuring them will only backfire. Trust them to notice and follow their hunger cues.
- **Don't give into food requests before and after meals.** The old saying is true that eating before meals can ruin someone's appetite, and it's a way for a child to "hold out" for their favorite foods. How often does a child pick at their dinner and barely eat, even saying they aren't hungry, but then an hour later, they are hungry again and want a snack? Make these boundaries clear for your child, and don't let snacks before or after sway your efforts.

It's OK if your child decides not to eat. Have your child join the family at the table, even if they choose not to eat. If they skip the meal, avoid offering an extra snack later unless it's part of their regular eating schedule. It's OK if they go to bed hungry; it's a natural consequence that helps them learn to eat during scheduled mealtimes. (Again, your own history of going to bed hungry may stir up strong emotions at this moment. If you can stick with the schedule, do so. If you cannot navigate the emotions, add an evening snack to the schedule so there is another time to eat after the meal.) Over time, this approach can help them understand the importance of eating when food is offered, even if it's just a small amount, like bread and milk. Keep practicing. Be consistent with these messages. Change takes time, and you are setting the stage for them to grow into a well-rounded eater. Following these tips can help you achieve the goal of your child feeling good about eating. You don't want every meal to be a struggle, and you want mealtimes to be pleasant and happy. Yes, at first when putting these changes into place, there may be pushback, griping, or eye-rolling about new foods, but if you parent with love and no pressure, your child can learn to like unfamiliar foods, be more in tune with their hunger, know when they are not hungry or are full, and overall participate in fun, enjoyable mealtimes with your family.

We recommend sticking to your plan as much as possible and rolling with the changes as needed. Life happens. When it does, adjust the plan, but also stick with your goal. If Tuesday night's tacos get bumped to Wednesday night because of a makeup basketball practice, allow for that flexibility. Have Wednesday night's sub sandwiches as a quicker option on Tuesday. You are still meeting your goal of cooking more meals at home. Flexibility keeps the goal in place best. Rigidity makes us feel like we failed when the plan shifts some. Rigidity with your goals may seem like the best way to stick with the plan, but it can also set you up to fail. Be flexible while staying focused on your goals, roll with the changes, and keep moving forward.

Provide the Foods Your Family Enjoys

Don't become too caught up in what you *should* be cooking. When cooking more at home, focus on the foods you know how to cook and the traditional foods your family enjoys. We want to remove judgment about our family meal choices. You can enjoy the foods from your family's history, background, and culture without guilt. You are doing your job as a parent when you feed your family what you have and what you know. Adding guilt about what you *should* be providing doesn't help anyone.

Eat Together

For more than 50 years, people have steadily been eating fewer meals at home. Fast food, ready-to-go meals, and frozen meals with high levels of sodium have made eating convenient when the evenings are busy. For families, eating out can make family meals easier because everyone chooses their own meal, there are fewer food arguments, and there are no dishes to wash, with the added benefit of tasty food!

Unfortunately, these tasty, quick meals may not be the best option for our bodies if they are eaten frequently. They are often less balanced in protein, grains, and fruits and vegetables and include a lot of added fat, sugar, and salt. Even if the description of the food is on the menu, you don't always know what ingredients are in the dish. By cooking at home, you know what is involved and can change it to be appropriate for your family's needs. When our team is interviewed, we are always asked the same question: "What is the one thing you want people to know to help their family be healthier?" Our reply is always the same: "Have more family meals together at home!"

Importance of Family Meals

Eating regular meals together as a family has benefits beyond a balanced meal. Children who eat meals with their families 4 or more times a week have better emotional, social, and physical health:

- Lower risk for disordered eating, drug and alcohol use, violent behavior, depression, and suicidal thoughts, as well as lower stress levels
- Healthier eating habits, including more fruits and vegetables and less fast food and sugary drinks
- Healthier weight and lower risk for excess weight as adults
- Higher self-esteem and better communication skills

Eating together is potentially one of our best times to connect daily as a family. We all need to eat, and if we can find time in our schedules to do it together, it provides an opportunity to talk for a few minutes and connect with each other. Phones down, forks up—enjoy! Your family table is where you make memories and establish the *how* of eating for your family. Finding balance in what you provide is key to helping children learn to eat a variety of foods, reduce food obsessions, and have a healthy relationship with food that extends into adulthood. Restricting favorite foods can lead to overfocus on those foods, sneaking or hiding of foods, or loss of control when gaining access to the restricted items. Your children are learning that your family cares about each other and shows it by taking time for each other.

Ingredient Household Versus Snack Household

In busy families, food needs to be readily available, but how it's stocked can make a big difference. A helpful concept to consider is the difference between an ingredient household and a snack household.

An "ingredient household" has fewer ready-to-eat foods. Instead, it includes items that require simple preparation, like

- Slices of cheese with crackers instead of prepackaged cheese and crackers
- Desserts made from scratch, such as homemade cookies or microwave s'mores (graham crackers, marshmallows, and chocolate)
- Quick-fix meals, which might include
  - A whole chicken in the slow cooker, which allows for the protein to carry over into 2 meals, such as rice bowls or a pasta bake
  - Easy sides, like carrot sticks, bread, or sliced strawberries
  - Weekend meals, like chicken enchiladas that provide leftovers for a weekday

On the other hand, a "snack household" focuses more on convenience and ready-to-eat options. These might include

- Frozen pizza bites
- Cheese-flavored crackers
- Potato chips
- Snack cakes and packaged cookies

While snack foods are convenient, they're often hyper-palatable because they are high in sugar, salt, and/or fat, which can make them more "craveable" and less nutritious. These foods are typically ultra-processed and may not support long-term health goals.

Finding Balance

It's important to strike a balance between ingredients and snacks. Families benefit from having both, that is,

- Grab-and-go snacks for busy afternoons
- Basic ingredients for preparing meals at home

As life gets busier, it's natural to lean toward convenience. Children may pressure caregivers to buy more snack foods because they're tasty and heavily advertised. But shifting toward more ingredient-based meals can lead to pushback.

Here are some tips to ease the transition.

- Keep both options available to support flexibility and reduce stress.
- Expect some resistance: you may hear "We don't have anything to eat" as your household adjusts.
- Don't eliminate all snacks; this change can feel restrictive and make those foods even more desirable.
- Plan ahead to prepare meals using ingredients you already have.

> ### What Is a "Relationship" With Food?
>
> When we say a *healthy relationship* with food, this means your child grows up enjoying a variety of foods, is able to listen to their body's hunger and fullness cues, and can eat without feeling guilty.

Making Family Meals Happen

School, activities, and jobs all make our schedules complicated, and having time to enjoy a meal together can be tough. We don't mean to put pressure on you, making you feel that if you don't have regular family meals together, you are harming your children. Absolutely not! The most important thing is the love and care you show your children. Having family meals can be part of that, and finding ways to adapt to that within your family will only make more opportunities for that love to shine through. Whether it's a Saturday brunch, an old-fashioned Sunday dinner, or breakfast on a Wednesday morning, make the family meal a priority. Find the right frequency of family meals for your home, whether that is every day or only on weekends. Here are some tips for how to get started when you are ready to add more family meals.

- Gather all family members when it's time to eat. Whoever is home will join the meal at the designated eating time.
- It doesn't matter where it is. We encourage eating at the table, but finding a place to eat together (with all electronic devices off) is key. Gathering in the living room or at a kitchen counter can work depending on where your family can get together best in your home.
- Invite children to help set the table. Involving them builds their investment in the activity.
- Have sit-down snacks together, when possible. Include children in planning snacks and enjoy these with them.
- Don't force someone to speak. Keep the space open for anyone to talk.
- Enjoy this time together with pleasant conversation about topics other than food. Try out meal conversation starters. Here are some examples.
  - What is your favorite family tradition and why?
  - If you could visit another country, where would you go and why?
  - What was the best thing about your day today?
  - Would you rather sing all day or dance all day and why?

- Try out "highs and lows" of the day (explained in Chapter 2, Parenting Through Structure and Love; see the "Encourage people to talk" list item). This is time to show support, empathy, and understanding. As a reminder, often teens just want to be heard, so rather than immediately jump in to give suggestions on any of their challenges, simply listen.

Turn Off Electronics

To keep meals about the food and people you're eating with, it requires turning off electronics. This includes tablets, computers, TVs, smartphones, handheld games, and any other device that will take a person out of the conversation or cause distractions. This allows us to be more in tune with what we are eating, to enjoy the food, and to notice when we get full (also known as mindful eating or intuitive eating). It also allows for conversation and interaction. Here are some tips to get started.

- Set a rule of "no electronics" during meals for everyone.
- Silence all electronics and place them into another room or into a box. An "electronics basket" was very helpful in our home for a while.
- Start slowly and build up. Maybe allow electronics for the first week and then institute the new "no electronics" rule. Consider giving a heads-up about when the rule will go into effect so there are no surprises when it does.

And don't forget to include your children in all aspects of the meal—include them in cleaning up after the meal, allowing for even more time together and teaching valuable lessons.

Diving Into the Conversation

In our clinic, we hear about conflicts over food in homes on a weekly basis. Concerns include when caregivers want their child's weight to improve and when children receive comments about eating less food, such as "Don't you think you've had enough? Maybe eat more of your vegetables first" or "Finish your salad before you get seconds of meatloaf." Without a doubt, comments like these usually don't get the result you are hoping for, and often they lead to hurt feelings, particularly in children who may be concerned about their weight. This type of change can be new for a lot of parents, particularly if their child has picky eating or they are worried about their child's weight. Here are some things to remember.

When we try to get our children to eat *less,* they

- Tend to eat more at other times of the day
- Sneak food or try to eat away from us so we don't see how or what they are eating
- Want to eat those foods even more

When we try to get our children to eat *more,* they

- Tend to eat less of the foods we are encouraging them to eat more of
- Become more selective with the foods they will accept
- Argue about the food more often, often negotiating

The cycle of pressure, as noted in Figure 6.5, shows how pressure on a child can quickly spiral out of control. The more pressure they receive from caregivers and outside influences, the more likely they are to develop the following concerns:

- Lower self-esteem
- Weight gain
- An unhealthy relationship with food and exercise
- Increased stress within the family

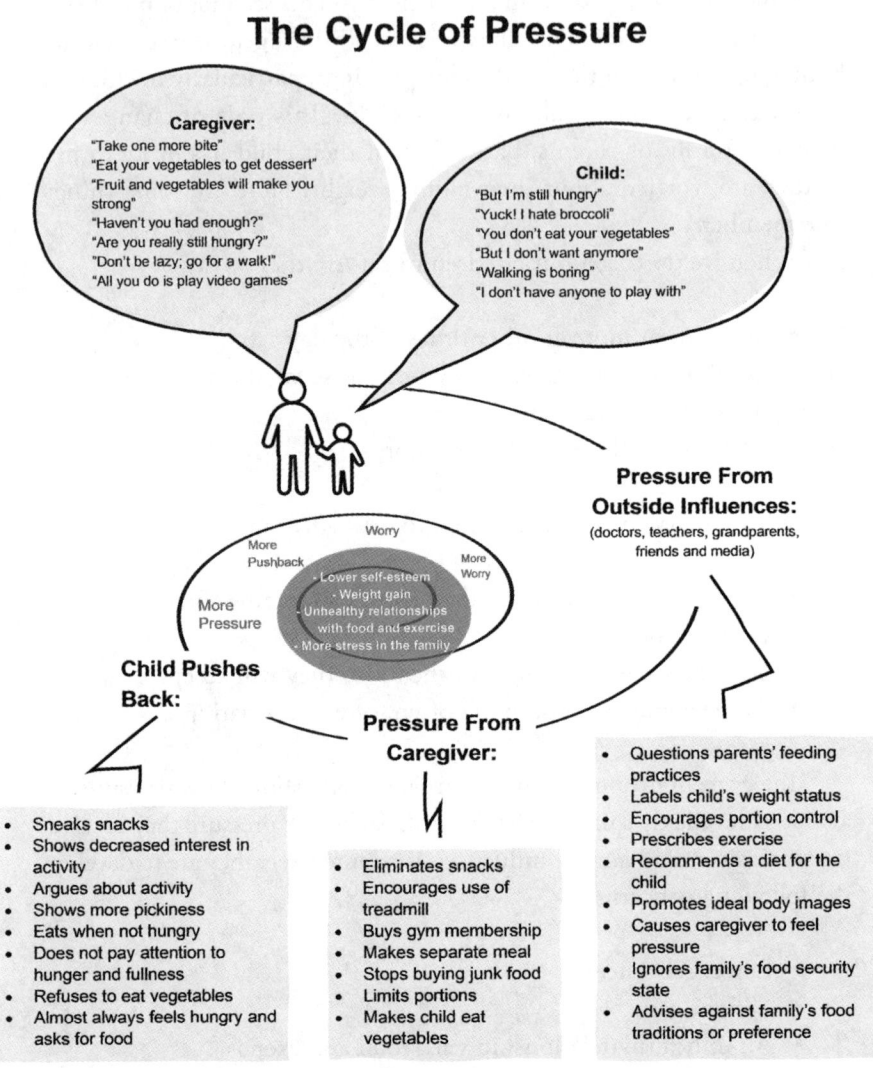

Figure 6.5. The Cycle of Pressure

Source: Derived from Dr Katja Rowell's "Worry Cycle."

Chapter 6 | Small Shifts, Big Impact: Transforming How Your Family Eats

Here are some things to remember.

- **Trust your child;** once they are on a schedule, their bodies will get what they need to grow. As Ellyn Satter recommends in her work, trust is essential. Trust lets children eat the amount that is right for them.
- **Stick to the meal and snack schedule,** even if your child doesn't eat what is being offered. Don't offer substitutes, as that teaches them they don't have to eat what is being offered and can increase picky eating.
- **Find something to talk about other than food.** For younger children who you suspect of not being hungry between meals, try redirecting them to another activity, such as playing a game or preparing their school items for the next day while they wait for the next mealtime.
- **Understand that children's appetites change.** Some days children will eat a lot and other days not so much. If we try to modify or control that with comments, pressure, and restriction, it will only interfere with their own internal hunger gauge.
- **Avoid pressuring children to eat less.**
  - Let your child decide how much to eat.
  - Allow additional helpings, if available, with no strings attached.
  - Allow your child to serve their own plate. For younger children, you can ask them how much they want on their plate.
  - Try serving the meal family-style, where the food is on the table so children can get more as needed.
  - Keep a neutral facial expression when you begin to worry about how much your child is eating.

Since we opened our program almost 20 years ago, we have heard families repeatedly say what a difference having family meals made. Children tell us the favorite part of participating in our program is spending more time together as a family (Yes, even the teenagers say that!). In particular, by removing the pressure from caregivers to be the food police, and creating that time to catch up with one another, these family meals can be quite a positive experience, which is why research has shown so many positive benefits from having regular family meals.

Putting Ideas Into Action

By now, you've heard a lot of practical ideas for how to eat on a schedule, cook more meals at home, and make time to eat together as a family. It's important to remember that you don't need to implement everything all at once.

- **Make realistic goals.** Think about what works for your family right now. For example, if you're in the middle of baseball season, cooking more meals at home might not be the best place to start. Choose goals that fit your current lifestyle.
- **Start small.** Ask yourself this: What small change could we make this week? No change is too small—every step forward counts.
- **Practice and be patient.** Change takes time. If this week didn't go as planned, that's OK. Start fresh next week. The key is to keep trying.
- **Celebrate successes.** Encourage each other when you make progress, even if it's just a small step. You're in this together and supporting one another helps build lasting habits.

We recommend choosing 1 or 2 habits to begin practicing in your home. Following are some simple options to start:

- Create a meal and snack schedule.
- Eat dinner together as a family.
- Turn off or put away electronics during dinner.
- Cook one more meal at home each week.
- Make a "Meals to Remember" list with your family.
- Begin eating breakfast most days.
- Choose snacks with 2 food groups for better nutrition.
- Serve one meal for the whole family most nights.

Chapter 6 | Small Shifts, Big Impact: Transforming How Your Family Eats

What happened to Liz? Liz decided to focus on the *how*. She knew what she wanted to do: have more home-cooked meals and eat dinner as a family at their kitchen table with no phones or electronics. In a stepwise fashion, Liz took the following actions:

- She hung a calendar on the refrigerator and sat all the boys down on Sunday to talk about the schedule for the week. They put as much as they could on the calendar—for example, hockey practice, school meetings, doctor's appointments, when they had to ride the bus versus when they could ride with friends.
- Next, she put on there the nights that made the most sense to cook a meal, eat leftovers, and order takeout. She included the boys in the discussion and negotiated whose turn it was to pick the restaurant that week. This actively gave the boys responsibility and defined their contributions, and they didn't feel like she was taking anything away from them.
- Each night, she had a "sous-chef" or an "assistant cook" (one of the boys) who helped her prepare dinner and set the table.

Next thing she knew, Liz was meal planning, including scheduling time to go to the grocery store, which she had never done before. Over the next several weeks, she added other things to the family meetings on Sundays, including setting bedtimes and creating lists of chores for the children to help her, and the boys added fun topics like picking movie nights. Liz didn't discuss these additions as changes; she started out by calling a meeting and discussing the weekly schedule, presented as "So we all know what is happening this week." The boys were excited when it was their turn to pick the restaurant for takeout night, and she even got their feedback on what to fix for dinner. Liz made only a few actual changes in *what* they were eating, but she slowly, and without great pomp and circumstance, made changes in *how* they were eating.

CHAPTER 7

Parenting Through Exercise and Physical Activity

Mitchell's family is really into a healthy lifestyle. His parents focus on feeding the family healthy meals, have set limits on TV and video games, and make sure everyone has an appropriate bedtime routine. His parents built a gym in their garage with a stationary bike, weights, and mats for yoga and stretching. Both parents work out almost every evening and are encouraging Mitchell to join them, but he never wants to, as he finds it boring.

At 11 years old, Mitchell instead likes to ride his bike to the park and meet up with friends and to play volleyball at school during gym class. Mitchell is bigger than other students in his class and has been teased a little bit about his weight. Since his parents eat healthy, they believe he gained weight because he doesn't get enough exercise, since he rides his bike for only a few minutes every day and volleyball doesn't cause him to sweat or breathe hard. The more they encourage or ask him to exercise with them in the home gym, the more he tends to pull away.

What are Mitchell's parents thinking and feeling? Why won't he be more active with the family? He's becoming lazy and doesn't try that hard to be more active. If he engages in more exercise, he will lose weight and classmates won't tease him anymore. He'll even learn to like it like they do.

> **What is Mitchell thinking and feeling?** He wishes they would leave him alone. He can tell what they think about him by how they look at him. He doesn't want to do their exercises—it's boring and he prefers his bike instead.

Authoritative parenting—the Structure and Love approach—applies to exercise and activity as well. Just as struggles over mealtimes and snacks can cause stress, disagreements, and even arguments, physical activity and exercise can also be a challenge. Or, more accurately, a lack of physical activity and an increase in sedentary activity are what can generally cause the most worry in parents. Much in the way that parents feel like they can be the food police, many parents feel like they are in a constant battle with their children to get them to move more.

Parents may find themselves saying something like the following statements without realizing they are forms of pressure and restriction (as explained in Chapter 2, Parenting Through Structure and Love):

- "Walk around the block, and you can have a piece of candy."
- "Play outside for an hour, or you can't watch TV."
- "You should be sweating, or you're not being active enough."
- "You need to be trying harder."
- "We are going for a walk even if you don't want to."

These words and expectations put pressure on our children, so instead of enjoying the activity, they grow to dislike it. As we discussed in Chapter 2 (see the Most Important Influences section), if we bribe children to eat their vegetables in order to earn dessert, they will begin to dislike vegetables and put even greater value on dessert. For activity, they may

- Put up even more of a fight and do less activity.
- Learn to be active only for a reward and not want to be active any other time.
- Begin to focus on what their parents think about their weight.
- Think, believe, or learn that specific activity is not fun.

Common Challenges to Being Physically Active

All children and families are different, and many things can get in the way of activity. Following are some challenges we have noticed over the years that interfere with children and families being active:

- Busy family schedules.
- Challenges with electronic use and social media.
- Lower interest in activity for the child and their family.
- Pain or discomfort with activity (eg, foot pain, back pain).
- Allergies, asthma, musculoskeletal conditions, or other health conditions.
- Limited opportunities near home (such as access to sidewalks, playgrounds, and parks).
- Limited transportation or money.
- Increased pressure to be more active.
- Caregivers can't participate because of health symptoms (eg, pain, breathing problems).
- Children and adults enjoy different activities.

You might relate to one or more items on the previous list. Adding more activity into our daily routine isn't always as simple as it seems, and it can be challenging for parents and children to make it a priority.

Busy Family Schedules

The reality of many families is that it is just downright hard to find time in the day to be active. This can be especially true on weekdays with work, school, and after-school activities keeping families busy. Just like with cooking at home, the key to increasing exercise is to plan ahead. It doesn't have to be the whole family together, especially as children grow older. Taking time to discuss activity time as a family at the beginning of the week may be a strategy that works for you.

You may also consider splitting the activity time up; it can be 10 minutes here, 20 minutes there. Smaller chunks of time can feel more manageable. It does not have to be a solid-hour block of activity. Too often, if we can't do an activity for 30+ minutes, we don't bother. I find that in the mornings when I get up to exercise, if I wake up late, pack my lunch, or send an email, and I find myself with only 15 minutes left, I skip the workout and just go in to work early. I've now adjusted to make do with the time I have, because any activity is better than none, whether it's 10 minutes long or 60.

Families have many competing priorities, and time can be tight. If you look at the weekly schedule and struggle to find time for physical activity, take advantage of where schedules overlap: some family members may choose to walk around the field while attending the practice of another child; children studying with a friend can schedule a walk break every 30 to 60 minutes, or they can walk to a friend's house to do homework.

If Monday or Tuesday is just too busy, schedule longer activity times on Wednesday, or even double up on weekends if that allows for more flexibility. Start where you are and slowly build activity into your week. Setting the goal higher than can be met may set you up for frustration and make you feel as if you failed. If starting with once a week is the most realistic, then that's what is right for you. Also, recognize that your family's busy schedule fluctuates; next semester or year might open up more, so do the best you can in the present moment and give yourself some grace.

Challenges With Electronic Use and Social Media

We often find that electronic use is one of the top reasons our children do not want to be active. For parents of younger children, the early years are an opportune time to develop a strategy of how your children will engage with electronics, including the household rules you set up regarding their use. For parents of older children and teens who may be concerned about the amount of their child's electronics use, you'll want to develop a strategy to implement rules and limits without getting into disagreements and hurting relationships. We often hear from parents and other caregivers in our program that once their children get used to taking their phones and devices into their bedrooms at night, it's an uphill battle to get them to stop, and the parents wish they never allowed their children to do that in the first place. Decide on the rules and regulations of electronics for your family as soon as you can.

Some families find it helpful to establish screen-free time. For your family, this may be right after your children get home from school and have their snack or right after dinner. By having this time away from screens, we often find children will be more open and able to participate in activity time.

Healthy Media Habits

The American Academy of Pediatrics (AAP) Center of Excellence on Social Media and Youth Mental Health has developed guidance for parenting around media use called the 5 Cs: child, content, calm, crowding out, and communication. Following are tips parents can use to support healthy media habits in their family:

- **Child:** Recognize that every child is different, and how they use media will vary. It can be educational, support an interest of theirs, and be a social connection. It can also contribute to poor mental health and expose them to violent or harmful content. Talk with your child about their media use and interests and how these may be affecting them.
- **Content:** The quality of what children are viewing and interacting with can vary widely. Find out what they are using different media devices for, and pay attention to how their use may be affecting them.
- **Calm:** Media use can elicit strong emotions in children, sometimes in ways that can affect their mood and attitude. Media use in the evenings can affect children as they try to fall asleep. Look for other outlets for children to calm down and relax before bed.
- **Crowding out:** Children and families may become engrossed in different media games or activities, which can lead to crowding out of other activities. Take time to discuss things your children and family enjoy doing, and make a plan for adding things back into your days that

don't involve screens. This can be helpful in setting limits for when media can be used and in planning for these other activities.
- **Communication:** The earlier you start discussing media use with your family, the easier it can be to navigate usage. If children are having difficulties, such as with school or friends, discussions of media use can be stressful and lead to arguments. Talk about the use of media early on and in positive or neutral ways and listen to their perspective on the ways they use media and technology.

For more information, check out the AAP Center of Excellence on Social Media and Youth Mental Health at www.aap.org/en/patient-care/media-and-children/center-of-excellence-on-social-media-and-youth-mental-health.

Lower Interest in Activity for the Child and Their Family

All children have different interests, and some simply find activities and sports completely uninteresting. The same goes for adults. So what is the best way to encourage physical activity if your child shows no interest? Model it yourself. Make it fun! It may be helpful to sit down together and discuss your interests (Figure 7.1).

Make Walking Fun!

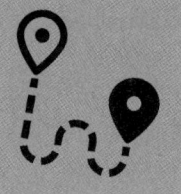

Go with a friend, listen to music or your favorite podcast, walk the dog, walk to a nearby store, call a friend or family member to catch up, or turn it into a nature scavenger hunt.

Family Activity Ideas

Place a check mark next to the activities your family enjoys. Add your own ideas in the blank spaces.

- ☐ Weight lifting, strength training
- ☐ Martial arts
- ☐ Gymnastics
- ☐ Running
- ☐ Dancing
- ☐ Twirling a hoop around the waist
- ☐ Walking in the neighborhood or at a park
- ☐ Tag
- ☐ Relay race
- ☐ Obstacle course
- ☐ Playing in the water, swimming laps
- ☐ Arts and crafts
- ☐ Games such as chase, tag, or hopscotch
- ☐ Using a jump rope
- ☐ Board games
- ☐ Playing on a playground
- ☐ Riding bikes
- ☐ Skateboarding, skating, rollerblading
- ☐ Volleyball
- ☐ Outdoor play, climbing trees, hide-and-seek

- ☐ Soccer
- ☐ Racket sports: badminton, tennis, pickleball
- ☐ Basketball
- ☐ Hiking
- ☐ Bowling
- ☐ Yoga
- ☐ 4 square
- ☐ Football
- ☐ Plastic bricks, cars, and other active toys
- ☐ Baseball/softball
- ☐ _____
- ☐ _____
- ☐ _____
- ☐ _____
- ☐ _____
- ☐ _____
- ☐ _____
- ☐ _____
- ☐ _____

Figure 7.1. Family Activities Ideas Checklist

Post the list of activities that your family checked off (that they enjoy) somewhere everyone can see, and when it's time to do an activity, choose from the list (Remember "out of sight, out of mind" from Chapter 2, Parenting Through Structure and Love?). It is easy to forget things you don't see, so posting lists can be helpful. Giving children a sense of ownership and control will frame the activity as fun rather than required. In other words, you want to make sure they don't see this as something they have to do because of their weight; rather, it is fun! And doing it with them will make an even greater impression.

Another approach to try if there is pushback is to make a list of the activities you want to do or try, and have your child make a list as well. Then see which ones overlap. This can be used to find mutual activities or to make a friendly trade-off, where the parent tries one of the activities their child likes (Figure 7.2) and vice versa. But be careful not to use this as a way to push an activity that you *want* your child to try and they have resisted previously, like running or an exercise class. Once you find what you have in common, that can be the first area to get started with.

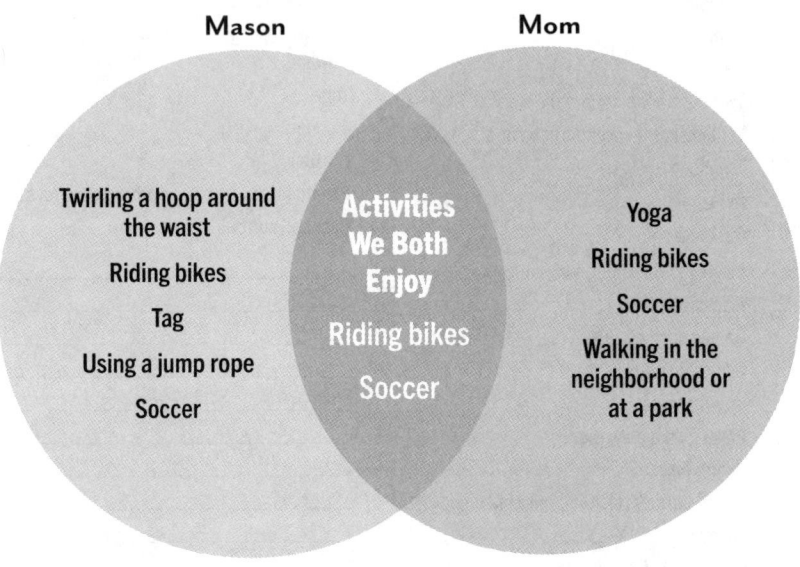

Figure 7.2. Overlapping of Family Activities

Pain or Discomfort With Activity (eg, Foot Pain, Back Pain)

Children's activity levels can be based on how skilled they are in certain movements. This includes basic, fundamental skills, also known as physical literacy, which includes throwing, catching, striking, jumping, running, kicking, agility, balance, and coordination. Each skill builds on previous movements, creating a strong foundation for physical activity, play, and daily life tasks. When a child struggles with any of these skills, it limits their ability to build the skills needed to participate in certain activities and sports as they get older. This can cause them to become discouraged and not want to participate, leading to a loss of confidence to be active. Ensuring regular time to play, be active, or just be outside and moving around, even with busy schedules, is one of the best ways to improve on basic movement skills. Children will naturally practice balancing, jumping, throwing, catching, walking, and running when playing with others.

Pain can also make it harder to master these skills, especially if a child is carrying excess weight. If your child regularly experiences pain during activity or movement, it could be worthwhile to see your child's health care professional or a physical therapist. Most of the time, as we now know with uncomplicated lower back pain and other health symptoms, moving more is what is needed, but make sure you confirm the pain is not from a specific condition first.

Find ways to move that don't hurt or are not uncomfortable and do these activities more often. If your feet hurt, try bike riding or swimming. If your back tends to hurt while playing basketball, try a different sport that doesn't use that particular part of your body. Modify whatever activity is causing the pain. I have a problem with my left shoulder caused by an old injury (the old injury being "growing old"), so I have modified my weight lifting to still use that arm but only do exercises that don't hurt or worsen the injury. After 1 to 2 weeks, try the uncomfortable movement again but for a shorter amount of time and in a way that doesn't hurt. For example, if walking causes foot or back pain, take a break from that and try biking, swimming, or bowling. After a break, try a shorter walk, maybe with a different pair of shoes or on a flatter surface, and build up to longer distances.

If your child is continually expressing pain or discomfort with exercise and activity, talk with their doctor to see if there is anything serious and if further exercise will make it worse. If there is nothing worrisome, pursue a different activity. Be aware if repeated expressions of pain or discomfort are getting in the way of being active, as these could be a sign of your child not wanting to do the activity (after you have determined there are no other problems). This could indicate that they feel pressure to be active, so backing off for a while may help. This is an important time to send the message "I still love and care for you—my feelings for you are not contingent on your exercising." Finding other ways to spend time with your child, such as playing board games, going shopping, or preparing a meal together, makes the message clear that your affection does not depend on them being active. In our experience, when you begin spending positive time with your children, that can lead to more active experiences, like walking, bike riding, or swimming.

Allergies, Asthma, Musculoskeletal Conditions, or Other Health Conditions

Health conditions can get in the way of children being active. Some of these challenges may cause movement delays or may be difficult to overcome, such as a broken leg or an inflammatory disorder. Many health conditions, such as asthma and diabetes, can be managed to an extent that they shouldn't significantly interfere with exercise and activity; but if they stop you or your child from being active, look into how they are being managed. Meeting with your child's health care professional to discuss this is very important, as they would not want these conditions to keep you and your child from being active. Sometimes there are other therapies that can be tried to manage the health condition and allow for exercise. For other health conditions, such as musculoskeletal or neurological diseases, meeting with specialists (adaptive exercise specialists, recreation therapists, or physical therapists) can be helpful in finding ways to be comfortable with activity.

Limited Opportunities Near Home/Limited Transportation or Money

Enrolling children in sports and driving all over town can be costly. Finding activities close to home can be a more budget-friendly option. It's perfectly fine to set aside time for fun activities inside or right outside your house.

Budget-Friendly Outdoor Activities

- *Obstacle course:* Use household items like chairs, ropes, or boxes to create a fun challenge. Ensure that what is set up or created is safe to navigate for children of all ages.
- *Nature scavenger hunt:* Look for specific leaves, rocks, or bugs in the yard.
- *Jump rope or hopscotch:* Try a jump rope or use outdoor chalk to create a hopscotch court. This is great for improving coordination and balance.

- *Walking or running:* If a walking or biking path is accessible near your home, this is an easy and inexpensive option. It can be even more fun when walking the dog, listening to music or your favorite podcast, or having a friend join.
- *Tag or hide-and-seek:* Search for classic games that children and caregivers can enjoy together.
- *Bikes or scooters:* If your child has either, riding around the neighborhood is a great way to be active.
- *Gardening:* Assigning chores to children to help with gardening in your yard or on a balcony teaches important lessons and can help save you time. Even pulling weeds or watering plants can be fun and educational.
- *Hiking:* This is a great way to see nature and get the whole family involved.

Budget-Friendly Indoor Activities

- *Dance party:* Play music and let your child dance around the house or wherever there is space.
- *Exercise videos:* There are plenty of free options online! Try kids' yoga, stretching, cardio, or body weight exercises.
- *"Keep it up":* Using a ballon, see how long your family can keep it off the ground while hitting it back at each other. This can also work as a game of indoor volleyball.
- *Active video games:* Find video games that get you moving, like dancing or sport games. While we often worry about children's electronic or screen time, there are many games that include physical activity and can be an outlet for children who may not enjoy sports or when weather prevents outdoor play.
- *Simon Says or freeze dance:* Find some classic games that require no equipment or money, as these are fun ways to improve listening skills and movement.
- *"Floor is lava":* This game involves someone saying, "The floor is lava!" Everyone jumps off the floor. If you touch the floor, you're out!
- *Homemade bowling:* Collect empty plastic bottles, then find a ball, any size, to use as a bowling ball.

Local recreation centers are also the perfect place to borrow equipment to use in their facilities. Keep an eye out in the summer! In our community, families that sign up can bowl for free all summer long, a local gym offers free memberships, and the city's parks and recreation department opens up its community centers with a rotating list of activities for children and families.

Increased Pressure to Be More Active

Increased pressure can be a big contributor to your child *not* wanting to be active. When we pressure our children to move, they tend to put up even *more* of a fight and do *less* physical activity. Even coaxing and bribing our children to be active can backfire. In these cases, they may even be less active than if they were doing it on their own. This pressure might look like "If you exercise for an hour, you can get an extra hour of video games tonight" or "If you run for half an hour, 3 times this week, I will give you $5."

Being pushed to be active is not fun for adults or children. Much like providing a single meal, and allowing children to decide which foods to try, give children different activity options and let them choose. When both my boys were in elementary school and I was on pickup duty in the afternoons, we had electronics-free time until dinner. I was so excited when I bought the latest yard game that everyone was playing, but my boys showed no interest in it. A few weeks later, when I told them they could pick the game to play during free time, they chose that game—the one they showed no interest in before! Likely, my pressure for them to play it turned them off, or they just weren't in the mood that day, but they were another day.

Don't focus on "exercise"; talk about activity as doing things the family enjoys, playing, and getting our bodies moving. Sometimes even just taking your child to the park can be the perfect opportunity for them to be active on their own accord. Even if they want to just sit on the bench at first, at some point, they will see you and others enjoying themselves, become bored, and want to join in. But it is perfectly OK if they continue to sit on the bench. The point is you have done your job in offering the opportunity. Let them decide how active they want to be. We know this can be frustrating, but keep modeling activity yourself.

As noted earlier, don't automatically assume that any pain or other concerns expressed during exercise are made up or not true. Take these concerns seriously by exploring them with your child's doctor before assuming your child is making excuses to get out of activity. Take steps to still spend quality time with your child to send the message of love and acceptance.

Caregivers Can't Participate Because of Health Symptoms (eg, Pain, Breathing Problems)

This is a difficult one, as health conditions can interfere with activity. For many adults, shortness of breath, mild joint soreness, or other discomfort can occur when they are new to an activity or exercise and it can be normal and expected. Be patient and consistent, engaging in amounts or the intensity you are comfortable with and stopping when you are not comfortable or there is pain. Engagement is the most important part, not necessarily the amount or intensity.

The most frequent situation we see is that a parent has a physical or medical condition that may shape the way they do activity with their children, such as using a wheelchair or having a chronic illness that affects their breathing, whether directly (the condition itself) or indirectly (eg, a hiking trail that is not wheelchair accessible). In these situations, do the best you can by, most importantly, supporting your child's activity, whether that is taking them to a park to play, arranging a playdate, or being a positive support to them when they are trying a new activity. Some of the most powerful words a child can hear are "I love watching you do…," which reinforces your support of your child, including that you are their biggest fan. Even with health conditions, keep a schedule with electronics-free or active time in place.

Children and Adults Enjoy Different Activities

When we enjoy an activity, it's natural to want to share that with others, especially our children. And it's the same for our children: they want to share a fun activity with us, especially if they get to show us how it's done ("Hey, Dad, watch me!"). But it's also natural for everyone in families to have different likes and dislikes and not want to do the same activity.

It's a balancing act for families to find joint activities to do together and allow for individual activities. As the parent, you most often are going to be the one trying out an activity with your child, even if it's not one that you enjoy. When spending time with my children, I have tried activities I don't enjoy as much, like a multiplayer video game or pickleball. But my children were thrilled for me to try it with them, and it gave me a better understanding of what they were doing and how they enjoyed it.

Even though you may try out their activity, don't necessarily expect them to do the same; they may be resistant to engage in your activity. They may see it as tricking them into exercise or as making a trade-off: "I tried your video game, so now you need to try tennis." But still offer anyway; they may appreciate the invitation, and your making them feel included, particularly if they see the activity as something the "adults" are doing. Finally, try out a new activity for the family; exploring it together may lead to an activity everyone enjoys, or even just one family member enjoys. My own family did this with disc golf. While we were trying to find a family activity that everyone enjoyed, disc golf eventually became the main sport and passion for my oldest son.

Battle Hymn of the Electronics

Caregivers and children are often at odds over the use of electronics. For children in bigger bodies, or if parents and children are concerned about weight, there can be increasing pressure to be more active. We hear quite frequently that parents believe that lack of activity results in their child's weight gain. Unfortunately, this can lead to strong assumptions or conclusions (eg, "He's lazy, and all he does is play video games," "I tell her to put her phone down and exercise," or "They would lose weight if they would just be more active and not lie around so much").

In a split second, concerns about electronics use and not enough exercise can rapidly turn into criticism and negative comments that cause conflict, hurt feelings, and damage relationships. What started out as a parent or caregiver wanting their child to be healthy—to develop strong bones, a strong heart, and strong lungs, which can come from regular exercise—leads to adults and children on opposite sides of a dispute over screen time and physical activity. We see pictures all over social media, and in books and magazines, of families doing fun activities together, which can make us quickly feel like failures when we argue with our teens over their phones and social media, when we would much rather be enjoying time together.

How Can We Avoid Disagreements Over Electronics?

Technology, video games, internet, smartphones, social media—they are all fun! Even we adults find ourselves easily distracted (as I write this chapter, I find myself reaching for my phone to check social media). When we watch our children use electronics and we stress over the exercise and activity they are missing out on, we often forget we didn't have this level and degree of technology at their age. Technology is a lot of fun and can be a strong draw from the activity and exercise that can build our children's mental and physical health. If you notice that electronics are getting in the way of your child being active, here are some suggestions on how to navigate it.

- **Explain the why.** Explain why you want to have this conversation about media and electronics, including the reasons why changes need to occur. Don't expect them to understand or agree, no matter how compelling or clear your argument, and listen without judgment. Discussing how devices or media are used is valuable. Teaching about misuse, online safety, and scams can lead to a lifetime of wise internet and technology use.
- **Establish tech-free time.** Rather than set limits on *the amount of time* spent on electronics and devices, focus on *how* the time is spent on electronics. In older teens, it can be difficult to set exact limits because of their growing independence and time spent away from home. The recommendations in the AAP Family Media Plan can help track these family rule changes. Establish tech-free times of day or tech-free zones, or limit to one screen at a time, such as watching a movie but not also scanning social media on a phone.
- **Listen and discuss boundaries.** Before setting up screen time boundaries for your home, listen. Let your child or teen say what times of day or which online activities are important to them. Allow for negotiation that not only helps you manage the expectations that are most important to you but

also creates space for your child's preferences. Their voice matters. You may be surprised by how much your child can set their own rules when given a calm time to discuss what is needed together. This conversation may start by conveying you are concerned about how tired you see your child in the afternoons, so to help them get more sleep, there will be some limits on devices at night. Then ask what your child thinks might help. You can offer options if they don't think of anything at first: "Phones will have to stay in the charger in a different room overnight, but what time should they go on the charger?" "In the time between school ending and bedtime starting, when is it most important to have time on the phone or a video game?" Your family's rule could be that phones are off after a certain time or that you interact with only one screen at a time. As caregivers, we need to model this. Most smartphone plans through your provider have settings through which an adult can turn off internet access at night or even shut down the phone completely. You provide the structure that screen time needs to change and provide the love by listening and responding to your children's opinions.

- **Outline expectations.** Once rules are established, write them down. It will clarify expectations if they are written down. Your child or teen can be responsible for this part. It will also help to discuss what happens when the rules are not followed. Family members can provide a reminder that phones and other devices aren't allowed at the kitchen table. If the phones are not turned off, phones will be put away for the rest of the evening.
- **Determine a start time.** Set a date in the near future (eg, 1 day, 1 week) for the new rules to take effect. There are likely many new family policies you would like to set up (eg, no phones or other devices in the bedroom, no electronic use an hour before bedtime, no devices during meals), but to avoid becoming overwhelmed, consider implementing one at a time.
- **Follow up.** Set up a time to discuss the policy again in the future, a few weeks after it is in place. This allows you to problem-solve if the change didn't "stick," including how to get back on track, or to praise the family on making it happen.

We understand change is not always that simple. Many, many parents struggle with these routine changes, and sometimes the changes aren't successful or they cause significant conflict between parents and children. Every caregiver has to weigh and balance the benefits of screen time boundaries with the risks for heightened conflict that can arise from making these changes. The AAP has a great resource for families on how to have these conversations, known as the Family Media Plan (www.healthychildren.org/mediaplan), where families can set priorities, make plans, and track progress.

Shaping Behavior

As you transition to practicing adjusted screen time use, it often helps to focus on adding in an activity, or planning something fun together, and not focusing on getting rid of something, like screen time. A strong way to ease out of old screen time habits is to find fun alternatives that occupy that time. It is easier to create time *for* something. It is much harder to focus on the absence of something. For reducing screen time, it is a smaller adjustment to start playing cards as a family instead of playing video games. This may not increase active time at first. Yet it teaches us how to leave sedentary activities for a short time and do another fun activity that allows for family time. Once the card games are established as a fun activity to do together, the activity can shift to something physically active. With the foundational habit of family card games after dinner, the family could try adding a family walk to some evenings instead of cards or before cards. The family could try a different game, such as charades, or another option, such as balloon volleyball, to transition to something more active. Practicing the habit of leaving one activity to join a family activity is important.

A note of caution: We often see parents set up a physical activity for their children to replace electronics time. Much like with having to eat your vegetables to have dessert, this can cause your child to dislike the activity because it's replacing something they really want (eg, phone, tablet, TV). This can be a form of the P & R Coin (see Chapter 2, Parenting Through Structure and Love, specifically the P & R Coin: Pressure and Restriction section), where children feel pressured into activity and restricted from their electronics. Take a neutral approach by setting up the schedule to have electronics time *and* electronics-free time. Go back to the list of activities they enjoy and have them pick from that. Or in the beginning, they may elect to do nothing…which can be therapeutic, but it will eventually lead them to seek out another activity. It may not be active (eg, reading), but it's the first step in limiting electronics use.

> ### Baby Steps Toward "Shaping"
>
> In the field of psychology, there is a process called "shaping" to describe a change in behavior that occurs in small steps. Each step toward the goal or behavior is a win. If I want to go for a walk before work in the mornings, I consider that I'm moving toward my goal by waking up in time to add the walk but not actually walking yet. The next step might be putting on my T-shirt and tennis shoes and stretching or warming up. I'm still on the path to my goal if I walk for 10 minutes instead of my goal of 45 to 60 minutes. This process may take me 2 weeks or 2 months.
>
> Recognizing that I am on track and making progress is how I can reach my goal. I congratulate myself for each action to encourage myself to keep moving forward. Another aspect of this shift in thinking is my mindset. When I view these small steps as how I expect to move forward, it means I am doing just fine. I feel successful along the path to the goal. If I instead view these small steps as failures because I am not meeting the goal yet, I may feel inadequate and am more likely to stop trying.
>
> We all need to feel successful and see that our effort allows us to reach our goal. Setting expectations—how we define our effort, how we label the effort—is part of the mindset that can get us to the goal. We focus on what we are doing and then we set steps toward the goal. This process establishes structure and does so in a loving way, while respecting how hard the changes can be.

Increasing Activity as a Family

Shaping can also be applied to increasing family activity, not just individual activity. If you want your family to participate in fun activities together, check out the following tips:

- **Brainstorm a list of fun activities to do together.** Much like with the "Meals to Remember" list (see Chapter 6, Small Shifts, Big Impact: Transforming How Your Family Eats), keep a list of activities your children like. With all that is going on in our lives, sometimes we forget about an old activity, game, or sport we once really enjoyed, so having it written down can jog the memory and get us to try it again.
- **Don't force any family members to do something they don't like.** This can be tricky when there are several children in the home, with different preferences. Taking turns and making compromises are valuable lessons for children to learn through this process.
- **Find age-appropriate activities and participate together.** We tell children "Go outside and play." This offers a great opportunity for children to entertain themselves. Also, be willing to skip your exercise time to spend it doing a fun game with your child.
- **Start with a low-intensity activity at first** (eg, throwing a flying disk) and then move toward activities that require more movement and coordination (eg, soccer, one-on-one basketball).
- **Find a place to be active.** This can be something simple, like a local park or recreation center, or identify space in your home that can be customized for activity. Move chairs around to play indoor soccer with a sponge soccer ball.

Much like with eating habits, model being active and practicing healthy use of electronics. Adhere to electronics-free time, participate in play-based activities with your children, and support their choices of games and activities. I've never enjoyed baseball growing up and don't follow it now, but both my children did, so I got my own used baseball glove so I could throw with them. Some caregivers face activity challenges because of health or musculoskeletal conditions, so do the best you can to model what you can. If you can't participate in the activity, be present and cheer them on. Your family will notice the effort you are making.

Building the Schedule

In addition to having positive effects on our health, regular exercise and activity also reduce stress, improve our mood, increase concentration, and help us sleep better. In trying not to pressure your child into an activity (eg, "You must exercise for an hour to play video games later"), focus on the schedule, as we've talked about before. As you build your schedule for the week, start to add aspects of tech- or electronics-free time, then add in activity time (but notice, we didn't say *exercise*).

- Put a schedule up for each day and the rest of the week. Expand the weekly meal and snack schedule to include other things, such as electronics-free time, homework, and physical activity or play. If a weekly schedule is a struggle, start with a family calendar, marking the day for a family activity.
- Depending on your child's age, set an activity time or an electronics-free time. Younger children will likely be more open to having "outside" time or family activity time, whereas a teen might be more open to negotiating tech-free time. Pull ideas from the activities list you brainstormed before, and add the ideas to the schedule. For older children and teens, you can institute this but in a low-pressure way. Have it on the calendar, invite them to participate without pressure, and invite their input on an activity during that time. It's a great time to play the "parent card." If they say, "Watch a movie," for activity time, explain why that activity doesn't cut it because it still involves a screen (scheduling a movie night for another time, however, is a great idea). But if they say, "Play a board game," do it without comment. It may still be a sedentary activity but doesn't involve technology or screens.
- Try splitting activity into small chunks of time (eg, 15-minute increments). Any amount of activity is great. The long-term goal is getting an hour of physical activity a day for children,

but they don't have to get it all at once. And that is not where we start. Start with a small amount of time and build.

Let Your Child Decide How Much (or How Little) They Are Active

Children are open to moving more when they are allowed to decide how active they want to be. A common scenario in our program is when teens try to find a physical activity they enjoy doing, so they don't dread having to do it. It's heartbreaking when the teen finally gets into a routine with an activity, like disc golf or walking, and then someone comments, "But that isn't vigorous or intense enough to count as exercise." It's here that I remind families that some of the healthiest people are gardeners. Although gardening doesn't get your heart rate very elevated, it does involve using a lot of different muscles, it's very relaxing, and people tend to do it for many years, even as they become older and less mobile. The important part is the step that has been taken to do physical activity and be in a routine of doing it. Once they choose their activity, do not make comments or provide suggestions. Support them in their activities and help them make time to do these activities.

When children are pressured to be more active, they

- May push back, causing conflict
- Tend to participate less
- May develop negative feelings toward activity

When we remove the pressure for children to be active, they

- Learn to enjoy activity
- Gradually start to find ways to be active on their own
- Will be more open to participating in planned family activities
- Are more likely to be active if the activity is something they enjoy and if others join in

Teenagers: Not Quite Children, Not Quite Adults

Adolescents often fall "in between," where they not only are less likely to do the free play that younger children enjoy but also may have hesitation to engage in other "adult exercise" activities, such as running, lifting weights, or going to the gym. Then again, some teens like doing outdoor games such as scavenger hunts or will train at a gym to hone sports skills. Luckily, many teens like to play sports, either competitively or recreationally. Sports have become very competitive and expensive to participate in, which can be prohibitive for many families. Over the past 20 years, many children who once enjoyed sports stopped participating in their middle and high school years because of the high levels of competition, cost of club leagues, and limited number of school teams. Regardless of their competitive nature, sports are still a great and fun way to stay active, at all levels of play. And there are hundreds of sports for children to take up, from pickleball to flag football to table tennis to geocaching (I admit, I had to look that up when my cousin said it was her favorite activity). If teens show interest in adult exercise activities, support that interest as best you can, but allow for trial and error. Don't buy a yearlong membership at a gym that your child may try for a while and decide is not for them. Several gyms allow children to join starting at age 12 years and offer trial memberships in the summer or over holiday breaks or have day passes. Explore less expensive options, such as free videos found online that can be watched at any time.

Balancing School and Homework to Include More Physical Activities

Parents and caregivers of school-aged children and teens know that homework is a daily task needing time and attention. From that very first tearful kindergarten drop-off, homework has been a piece of the daily time management plight for many parents. Trying to complete assignments in the after-school and before-bed hours, while adding activity, music lessons, clubs, religious activities, or team sports for one or many children, gets to be a calendar nightmare. Caregivers are rushing to get children to activities with the necessary gear. A meal must also be cooked or purchased. Homework can be a brief reading practice or a multiple-hour effort to complete an essay.

There is no simple answer to how to find balance with activities, homework assignments, and the limited hours available outside the school day. Some households find that simpler is easier, so they limit the outside activities. Some households find that staying busy works better, so they find ways to juggle multiple commitments. Others prioritize family time, or care of their bodies, or volunteering or academics. Priorities change as your children and teens get older. You will need to make adjustments at each stage to find the balance available at that time.

Families cannot add more hours to the week, but there are ways to capitalize on your time. From our experience working with thousands of families, and in our own busy families, we have found there are 2 ways to do so:

1. **Family Meeting:** This encourages the ever-important key to a happy and healthy family—communication! Touching base once a week, where all of you focus on everyone's schedules, can be very powerful. It lays out everyone's schedule, reveals ways to help each other get to where they need to be, and prevents last-minute scrambling. It also builds collaboration and investment of your family team in decisions made by all family members together. Family meetings are covered in Chapter 3, (Not) Talking With Your Kids About Their Weight (see the "Family Meeting" box).
2. **Weekly schedule:** Writing things out is the best way to identify where to fit in activities. This prompts communication and becomes the hub for everyone to check for what is happening daily. It can also help build in downtime for children and parents, where they can recharge for school and work.

Spending time with your teenager is important to you, and you want to find some activities in the day to spend with them; talking through how your day is scheduled, and where you spend your time, can be a great first step to finding 30 minutes to an hour to spend together as a family.

What happened to Mitchell and his parents? Mitchell's parents became more and more frustrated with him not being active. Volleyball season was coming to an end, and the weather was getting colder, so he wasn't riding his bike as often. This worried his parents even more, who tried everything they could to get him exercising: they began buying more fitness equipment, hoping he would like it; hired a personal trainer at the gym; and offered to increase his allowance for every hour of exercise he got during the week.

Unfortunately, this only made Mitchell feel worse about himself. He felt like a disappointment to his parents and became angry with them for pushing him so much. He now calls his parent's exercise routine "stupid," and when he has electronics-free time, he sits and reads magazines. If his parents mention exercise, he becomes angry and goes to his room. He now has no desire to play volleyball next year.

Mitchell's parents decided to "push the reset button." They all met with a family counselor, who was able to help his parents understand his feelings and to help him understand his parents' feelings as well. Their fear of him not getting exercise, gaining weight, and developing unhealthy habits was overshadowing their relationship with him. They began to understand that they were making him feel bad and that pushing him was not going to work. Now they set up time every week to do something he wants to do, without comment or criticism, and are having very positive times together. He has even chosen to go on a bike ride with his parents once a month, as long as he is able to decide when he is done.

CHAPTER 8

Picky Eating and Other Nutritional Challenges

Robin is always cooking 2 meals for dinner: one for her grandson, Jaylen, who has picky eating, and one for Jaylen's grandfather and herself. When he was a toddler, he refused to eat what they were eating and asked for a snack right after the meal. Robin worried he was not eating enough, so she gave him his favorite food of macaroni and cheese and chicken tenders most days after the family meal ended. Robin knew that this may not have been the best tactic to get him to eat more, but she did not know what else to do. She did not want to force him to eat his broccoli or make him sit at the table for hours until he finished the food he wouldn't eat. She had to do this when she was growing up. As Jaylen entered elementary school, he snacked all day long and he got upset when she said no to his snack requests. Instead of eating at mealtimes, he had the habit of snacking in between meals, where he could enjoy his favorite foods, like chips or crackers. As he grows older, Robin is worried he isn't getting enough nutritious foods, so she begins to hide vegetables in dishes she makes for him, but when he figures it out, he gets even more selective with what he eats (and becomes distrustful of her cooking). As Jaylen eats fewer and fewer foods, Robin is desperate, even offering him candy if he eats certain foods.

What is Robin thinking and feeling? She is frustrated over the inability to get him to eat foods she serves him. She imagines raising him to be a balanced eater like her and avoiding junk food. She believes she must keep pushing, encouraging, and even tricking him to eat vegetables so he can stay healthy. She also feels embarrassed about how picky her child is, having to pack food for him on playdates and knowing he is eating the same lunch every day at school. And finally...she is stressed! When she tries to do something about his picky eating, it always becomes a battle and the meals are miserable. She does not want him to be hungry, so in the end, she gives in.

What is Jaylen thinking and feeling? He is stressed too. Every meal, his grandma pressures him about what he is eating. He wishes she would just let him eat what he wants!

Considerations for Eating Behavior

While we try to understand children like Jaylen, who have more selective eating, it may be helpful to consider the myriad factors at play. Similar to how I have talked about eating behaviors in typical family meal situations, Table 8.1 lists some situations or conditions that may alter eating behaviors, appetite, activity, and weight.

If you or your children currently struggle with any of these considerations, or do so in the future, this chapter provides some suggestions for following a predictable eating schedule and maintaining trust around your child's eating while making the necessary food changes to live a happy, healthy lifestyle.

Table 8.1. Situations/Conditions That May Alter Eating Behaviors or Appetite

Possible Situations/Conditions	Nutritional Impacts
Neurodivergence • Autism spectrum • Attention-deficit/hyperactivity disorder	Sensitivity to texture, taste, or smell → selective eating Medications may suppress appetite during the day, and/or medications may increase appetite. Impulsivity → difficulty with mealtime structure Risk for avoidant/restrictive food intake disorder Changes made too quickly often not tolerated Preference/comfort in sameness and routine for foods and meals → selective eating
Medical Conditions[a] • Gastrointestinal disorders (Crohn disease, celiac disease) • Food allergies/intolerances • Type 1 and 2 diabetes • Irritable bowel syndrome	Specific foods must be avoided or limited. Medications can override hunger/fullness cues. Disrupted meal patterns
Parental Food Needs/Recommended Diets • Medical conditions affecting parental intake (eg, bariatric surgery, GLP-1 agonist use) • Diets, like vegetarian, vegan, gluten-free, keto, or weight loss meal replacements	Specific foods must be avoided or limited. Medications affect hunger/fullness cues. Parental decreased hunger → limited meal prep Parental avoidance of "bad" foods at home
Mental Health[a] • Anxiety, depression • Emotional eating • Avoidant/restrictive food intake disorder; anorexia nervosa; binge-eating disorder; other specified feeding and eating disorders, including night eating	Overeating or undereating Eating off schedule Guilt from using food for comfort Restriction or purging for weight control Selective eating

[a] Partial list. Many conditions require guidance by a registered dietitian, a therapist, or a pediatrician.
Source: Dara Garner-Edwards and Melissa Moses.

Picky Eating

On the surface, picky eating in children should lead to poor weight gain. Yet it is also strongly associated with excess weight gain. Think of picky eating as a continuum from disliking green vegetables to eating only 6 foods total. It is a really tough challenge. It sneaks up on you, it is hard to predict or prevent, and, when you do try to change picky eating, it seems to get worse! What gives?

There isn't a ton of research on what causes picky eating, or "food fussiness," as some researchers call it, but we know quite a bit about how children develop their taste buds. Children receive most of their nutrition from breast (human) milk or formula from birth until around 6 months of age. From 6 months to 1 year, they slowly transition to getting more of their nutrition from solid foods. By 1 year of age, they are likely receiving most of their calories from solid foods, which coincides with their transition to table foods. But they don't fully jump into what their family is eating. That is because their ability to bite and chew some foods is not fully developed, so parents have to adjust textures and cut up food to minimize the choking risk. From 1 to 2 years of age, they slowly transition more to eating what their parents make. From then on, depending on the child and age, children can typically eat what we eat.

If only feeding children was that easy.

Children are very curious about smells, textures, and colors when they transition to table foods. Mostly, they will be curious about foods their parents and others eat, so this transition is a great time to model eating for them. Apart from eating, children pick up so much just from observing. At a young age, they will mimic what their parents do, particularly in important milestones such as language development. As they grow older, children continue to pick up habits and behaviors of their parents and, in their teen years, from their friends and peers. Modeling balanced eating habits is incredibly important.

Family meals with new foods allow your child to observe you eating a variety of foods. Providing those same foods for your child creates an environment of exploration. It can be a full sensory experience that they enjoy with their hands, nose, mouth, and even ears as they hear crunchy foods. Particularly around 2 to 3 years of age, children's eating is heavily influenced by others (eg, parents, caregivers, peers) as they independently feed themselves during meals. So this is an ideal time to expose children to new foods and textures. Children's typical behavior around 2 years of age includes their desire to pursue independence, which results from their rapidly progressing verbal and motor skills. Because they can't always accurately express themselves, they often become more and more frustrated, which can result in outbursts or meltdowns.

While their interest in foods and tastes may increase, their behavior can have an impact on what they want or don't want to eat. This is where you may see "food regression," where children suddenly stop eating foods they previously ate regularly. All of us have stories of a food our children ate all the time and then suddenly stopped eating with no explanation. It may be a change in taste and preference, but more than likely, it's a way to establish their independence. They now have a growing awareness that they can decide what goes into their mouth. The more we try to squash their independence by forcing non-preferred foods, the harder they push back to do it their way.

Developing Food Preferences

In her wonderfully written and thoroughly researched book *First Bite: How We Learn to Eat*, Bee Wilson covers how people develop food likes and dislikes. While some people believe food preferences and picky eating are driven by genetic makeup and personality, she shows how our food preferences are actually driven primarily by our environment and, in a sense, are a learned behavior—for example, how often we are exposed to a food, how pleasant the exposure was, who in our lives is eating and enjoying the food, and how familiar the food is.

Our family, culture, and experiences of food will be the biggest drivers of what foods we eat. As she says in the book, "The main way we learn to like foods is by simply trying them." As a caregiver, you can increase the likelihood of your child becoming a balanced eater through consistent exposure to a variety of foods.

Between 4 and 7 years of age, children enter their "picky stage," although a more accurate term is *food neophobia,* where they fear new foods. This is different from *picky eating,* which is liking only certain foods or not eating a wide variety of foods. Food neophobia is not wanting to try or eat foods you aren't familiar with. We all have experienced this to some extent; depending on where you live, your culture may involve routinely eating grasshoppers, offal, or hot peppers, but these are not typical foods in my culture. In fact, one study showed that most foods people say they don't like are ones they've never even tried! For caregivers, differentiating between burgeoning picky eating and food neophobia is not that important. What is important is to know this is normal and occurs in many, many children.

What Am I Eating?

On a work trip to San Antonio, TX, our hosts ordered a bunch of different foods for us to try, and I fell in love with a warm, homey stew they served, menudo rojo. I was about halfway through when I asked what the meat was in the stew, and they told me: tripe! (If you don't know, *tripe* usually refers to the stomach lining of cows or pigs.) I was *thoroughly* enjoying it until I learned what it was, but suddenly I didn't want to eat it anymore. Why? Should knowing menudo rojo had tripe in it have affected my enjoyment of it? It did, unfortunately. I took a few minutes, thinking about how people develop their tastes and preferences and seeing my colleagues enjoying it so much. I focused on how much I enjoyed it, and not where tripe comes from, and continued eating (and loving) it. This was a positive lesson on how mental blocks, preconceived notions, and familiarity with foods affect our preferences and tastes.

What's a parent to do? In short, offer variety, but don't force it. Forcing backfires in a grand power struggle. It's important to note that there are key things we cannot force our children to do: eat, sleep, and go to the bathroom. For all these behaviors, we can teach our children and provide the right environment and opportunity, but ultimately, the child is in control of these functions. How we wish we could have made our children sleep when we needed them to! How many "curtain calls" did we sit through when they weren't tired, but it was bedtime, and they requested a drink of water or another goodnight kiss or another check under the bed? Parenting takes fortitude.

To guide an older child with picky eating through trying more new foods, I recommend encouraging the same behaviors you would in any child starting at age 1 year to prevent picky eating. Adhering to the following 6 steps is how to remove pressure around the picky eating. Remember that pressuring backfires in so many ways. The same is true for picky eating. The more we pressure children to eat vegetables or new foods, the fewer vegetables or new foods are eaten. Let's take a closer look at these steps.

1. Continue to offer meals and snacks on a schedule.

Offer 3 meals and 1 to 2 snacks at set times. For children with picky eating, snacking can be tricky. Sometimes snacks fill children up before dinner or can make up for what children didn't eat at dinner. Either way, snacking can lead to them being less hungry at mealtimes or learning they don't need to eat what's served at dinner. By not allowing eating outside scheduled times, you set your child up to be more successful with trying new foods. An old saying, of which a version shows up in the classic novel *Don Quixote,* is "The best seasoning is hunger."

2. Consider timed snacks.

If your child arrives home from school around 3:00 pm and dinner isn't until 6:00 pm, offer a filling snack when they get home. A snack with 2 food groups, like cheese and crackers or apples with peanut butter, can help hold them over until dinner. If they ask for food right before dinner, remind them what time dinner is. If they ask for a snack right after dinner, let them know it's not time to eat again yet. After-dinner eating can mean a few different things: they didn't eat much at dinner and therefore aren't full, they are bored and want to eat for entertainment, or they are angling for something besides a meal; after all, snacks are typically crunchy, salty, or sweet. Don't worry, your child will be OK if they eat very little or refuse dinner. Missing one meal is difficult and they will feel hunger. This teaches them that next time, they need to come join the family for dinner. When eating times are predictable, bodies adapt and become hungry just before scheduled meals. This provides the best environment for a family member with picky eating to be as ready to eat as much as possible. Feeding children on a schedule, giving them a chance to be hungry before the next meal, keeps them in sync with their hunger and nutritional needs. As long as they are growing well and steadily gaining weight, fluctuations in their appetite from day to day or meal to meal are not an issue. Remember the parenting types in Chapter 2, Parenting Through Structure and Love (see the Scientific Approach to Parenting section)? Encouragement, reminders to eat, and pushing of certain foods are all strategies that may lead to a few more bites in the short term, but in the long run, your child won't learn to enjoy new foods.

3. Continue to eat together for meals.
For parents, it is just as important for the family to eat together when there is a family member with picky eating as for any other situation. Children who are selective about their food need the opportunity to observe others enjoying a variety of foods. If a family member is eating a new food, the child is seeing the color and shape of the food, smelling the food while it's prepared, and observing the family member potentially enjoying the new food. A child with picky eating needs these experiences to become more comfortable with a new food. After positive exposure to others eating the food, the child may want to explore the new food as well. This may involve smelling the food; leaving the food on the plate but not eating, licking, biting, and then spitting out the food; or eventually tasting the food by dipping it into a favorite sauce like ketchup. Your child can know that it's OK to put the food into their mouth and be allowed to politely spit it into a napkin if it is not tolerable. Having this safe escape from the experience of an unpleasant texture or overwhelming flavor is necessary. They are allowed to choose whether or not to try all the foods, without comments about how much was eaten or what wasn't eaten. Modeling balanced eating behavior (if you make a big deal out of not liking a food, they will also pick that up over time) is going to have an impact.

4. Continue providing one meal for everyone to eat.
By including at least one food in the meal that you know your child likes, they will always have a safe food. This is a food they can eat, even if it is the only part of the meal they put onto their plate. It provides security,

a way to ease the stress of the meal. The same is true for allowing safe ways to try a new food: look first, smell, lick, and taste. These simple options remove the power struggle over what they choose to eat. We can also provide new ways to try foods by cooking in a different way. Having broccoli steamed, roasted, raw, or sautéed with a sauce offers very different flavors and textures. Adding condiments such as ranch dressing, ketchup, or cheese is allowed without concern if it provides a flavor that eases your child into exploring the broccoli. If your child doesn't choose to eat from the meal provided, do not offer a backup food. When the chicken, potatoes, and green beans aren't eaten, you have done your job by offering food at the time and place you determined. Your child decided not to eat. It is not necessary to then offer a bowl of cereal or make chicken nuggets. What does your child learn if this is done? Your child learns that if they refuse the food offered, they will still get a preferred food instead and learn to eat only favorite foods. By our continuing to provide a single meal for everyone, children are exposed to more variety and learn to eat the foods offered to them.

Looking At Versus Tasting Food

Fifteen times! That's right, approximately 15 times. That is the number of times a caregiver is recommended to offer a food to a child until they accept that food. The suggestion comes from a classic study that explored looking at versus tasting a food to reduce food neophobia. Note that the key word is *offer,* not *pressure* or *force,* so offer it on the plate or table for them to choose to eat if they want. Offer it over and over at different meals with no pressure to taste it. Don't make a big deal about it and don't let that food get labeled as a food they don't like. Don't rush to say, "Tim doesn't like that." Just allow your child to not eat it. You never know when they might finally try it again, or they may try it when prepared in a way they have never had before. I used to steer clear of the beloved southern staple pimento cheese, but then one day, it was served as a topping on a hamburger, and voilà! I was in love, after disliking it all my life!

5. Invite your child to be involved in the process.
When we include our child's input in the planning of meals and snacks, they learn that we want to respect their preferences. They learn that they are important and that food planning includes their needs. This can be further communicated by allowing children to explore the grocery store. Trust them to help select new foods to try as your budget allows. They might also want to help with gardening if growing foods is of interest to your family. Including our children in the cooking gives them the knowledge and skill set of how to prepare the food. Often when children help, they are more likely to taste the food being cooked. These steps help introduce them to new foods, let them know you are considering what they prefer, and may help them be more open to trying what they helped prepare. This is also an opportunity to continue modeling desired behavior. If your child helps plan dinner and they ask for chocolate cake for the whole meal, it's appropriate to say, "That's a yummy dessert. We can plan to have chocolate cake for your dad's birthday Friday. But let's pick something else for dinner tonight."

6. Learn to trust your child.
Children will feed themselves what they need to grow (as mentioned in Chapter 2, Parenting Through Structure and Love; see the "Dr Clara Davis: Changing How We Look at Children's Diets" box). The amount of food they eat can also evolve. You have likely seen this shift in your own children: they pick at their plates for breakfast and lunch and then eat a huge supper. Or for a couple of days, they don't seem to have much of an appetite and then eat as much as you do for a day. Allow your child to decide how much or how little to eat of foods provided. Allow your child to decide what foods go onto their plate. This demonstrates your trust in their eating. Let food remain on the plate without them having to eat it or taste it. Often when they put a new or unfamiliar food onto their plate, it is the first step to tasting it. They may or may not taste the food the first time they allow it on their plate. An unfinished plate is allowed, versus the tradition of making people "clean your plate."

Messages about food trust often go deeper than we realize. When we negotiate for children to have one more bite of a vegetable before dessert, we communicate that vegetables are a necessary evil required to earn dessert. It is important to remove this food hierarchy. If our children try a new food, they may need a safe way to escape the experiment. Tasting certain foods may be overwhelming. It is OK to provide the option of spitting the food out politely into a napkin. The food was tried, disliked, and removed. Move on and keep enjoying the meal together.

Praise and cheerleading can also feel like pressure to children. Don't praise them when they try a new food, as this type of praise is an indirect form of pressure, with the assumption that they have to keep eating to be in your good graces. Keep all comments about food neutral. When your child eats a bite of broccoli, there is no need to give this any attention. Inside, you are turning cartwheels. Outside, remain calm and cool. If your child comments, you can affirm that yes, you saw they ate their broccoli and you also like broccoli. The goal is for your child to try new and unfamiliar foods on their own and continue to try them based on natural curiosity and exploration. Praising eating in any form insinuates to your child that you want them to eat more of that food and can perpetuate the power struggle as they assert control of eating by returning to food refusal. When a new food is eaten, we talk about our day and let the eating continue. We are not to comment about what is eaten or how much. This helps them be more open to trying because the pressure is removed.

What Does Picky Eating Have to Do With Weight?
You might consider these lessons a child and family version of intuitive eating, letting children be in touch with their hunger—without adults interfering with it. This is authoritative parenting, taking the first step in breaking tension or control of a child's eating, putting them in control, but in the framework of the meal schedule. This approach sets them up to develop healthier eating patterns, allows them to maintain a healthy relationship with food and eating, and overall works to prevent excessive weight gain, and it even helps those children who are struggling with not gaining enough weight.

When attempting to convert picky eating into a more open mindset, avoid the following tactics:

- **Pushing or pressuring** a child to try a food will almost always backfire. The more pressure that is applied, the more likely it will be a negative experience. As I alluded to in the Picky Eating section earlier in this chapter, in Madagascar, Mexico, and other countries, eating insects is common and even a delicacy. Now imagine someone making you eat one (assuming you've never had one before); just building this thought up in the mind is enough to make some people gag. You may eventually try one but do so on your own time and because it doesn't seem so different anymore. Encouraging children isn't as noxious as pushing but is still a form of pressure. It can also lead your child to try the food only to gain praise and acceptance by you, so they don't learn to eat and enjoy the food on its own.

- **Bribing** children will also have the opposite effect over the long term. Promising a treat if they eat their vegetables (eg, "You can have a chocolate chip cookie if you eat your brussels sprouts") results in something called the *overjustification effect,* which means a child will be driven to eat the food only to earn a reward. For the example of dessert (chocolate chip cookie) for the vegetable (brussels sprouts), your child will label the vegetable as something not worth eating on its own and only to be consumed to receive a sweet. Holding the dessert as the reward sets up a hierarchy where certain foods must be endured to be able to eat the better foods. We want to limit giving a cookie even more power and elite status than it already has.
- **Doing nothing** and continuing to feed your child only the foods they want, without taking steps to broaden their palate, is likely to enhance their picky eating. There are instances where children can outgrow their pickiness, as we all know adults who talk about having picky eating as children, but that may not always happen. Take a proactive approach by setting up pleasant meals where your child knows their job is to eat from the foods served to them.
- **Tricking or deceiving** our children is a common trap we can fall into when our children begin avoiding fruits or vegetables. Examples are slipping in foods or hiding vegetables in their meals, trying to make food fun so they will eat. These tricks take a lot of work, and in the long run, they are not effective. In the short term, offer more nutritious food to your child, but the long-term goal is to serve food in the hope that it will open

your child up to new food experiences, where they will eventually grow out of a picky eating or food neophobic stage. As the parent, stick to your schedule and feeding principles and you'll save time, money, and a whole lot of stress.
- **"No, thank you" bites** is a concept that was popular in recent years, with a goal of trying to ensure that a child tries a bite before deciding they don't want any. The thought was that they still experienced the food and would maybe like it. Being forced to take bites, even small "No, thank you" bites, is a form of pressure that will backfire in the long run and won't accomplish our goal of exposing children to new and different foods and tastes. Children seek independence and autonomy, particularly around their foods, so let them try foods at their own pace.

Trust your instincts as a parent or caregiver. If you are concerned about your child's eating, talk with your child's doctor.

Autism Spectrum

Children on the autism spectrum often have sensory issues (sensitivities to taste, textures, or smells) that can complicate feeding and eating. These sensitivities may cause foods to be significantly aversive. In some cases, foods are used as a reward or part of a behavior management program, and children then become driven toward that food. Many children on the autism spectrum have a strong preference for routine and predictability, and they may have meltdowns if desiring a food and it is not provided. The desire for routine and familiarity can lead to children eating a narrower selection of food or being classified as picky. Further, some medications, such as atypical antipsychotics or antidepressants, can cause increased hunger and weight gain.

If your child is neurodivergent with issues related to taste, texture, and selective eating, first start with their pediatrician, or a specialized program for children on the autism spectrum (developmental and behavioral pediatrician, psychologist, or therapist specializing in this area), to discuss options. There are occupational therapists or speech therapists who can provide guidance and support with eating challenges.

Whether your child is young with no challenges related to food or is an adolescent who has a meltdown if they don't receive their favorite snack on demand, the Structure and Love approach can help (see Chapter 2, Parenting Through Structure and Love), although it's not easy, it's unlikely to give quick results, and the victories may occur less often. It can be hard to dissect the challenges involved, whether your child has a texture or taste aversion, increased hunger related to medications, or an increased focus on food, as either a reward or the innate drive to eat. Many aspects of setting up a structure around eating, avoiding getting into conflicts over food, and not pressuring or restricting can be of benefit for children on the autism spectrum. It may need to take longer to build a structure around eating, and you may focus on setting up schedules and appropriate rules for meals for a longer time, knowing that down the road, you can make a change to the foods being served (as Ellyn Satter says, the "what" of eating) as you navigate different reactions to the change. Setting up the structure would complement working with an occupational or speech therapist around texture issues or working with your child's care team around medications that could be increasing hunger.

Figure 8.1 is adapted from expert committee recommendations on addressing weight in children with autism and provides practical strategies to support healthy habits for children and their families.

For more than 20 years, we have worked with hundreds of children on the autism spectrum and their families, and every family is different. From our experience, when it comes to issues around eating and activity habits in children on the autism spectrum, the most common word we hear is *struggle:* struggle between parent and child over food, hunger, picky eating, electronics, and lack of physical activity. As children begin to gain weight, parents begin to hear comments such as "You need to feed more fruits and vegetables," "You need to limit portion sizes," "You need to get him more active," and so on. Of course, caregivers want all these things, but these are *way* easier said than done, as even small changes to the routine or food served can cause a meltdown or make the child stressed and unhappy. Directly trying to change these things can easily lead to conflict, arguments, hurt feelings…in short, it's a struggle. A common sentiment we hear is "It's just not worth it" as parents feel like giving up.

Balanced Eating	Physical Activity	Sedentary Activity
As able, involve children in planning and shopping for meals and snacks.

Keep language around food, meals, and eating habits positive.

Increase structure around mealtimes: display meal/snack schedule, and remove electronics and media.

Remove pressure from meals: offer new foods repeatedly to increase familiarity but without pressure to try.

If textures are a challenge, modify the texture in new foods.

Do not use food as a reward.

Work with school, child care, and in-home support staff to support what you are doing, particularly in having nonfood rewards (eg, activity, special privileges). | Include active family time in the daily and weekly schedules.

Include children in household chores, as able.

Work with the school on your child's individualized education program to include physical activity or adaptive physical education. | Increase structure around use of electronics and screen time, including on daily and weekly schedules.

Limit use of electronics and screen time as a reward or a break from caregiving.

Keep electronics out of bedrooms.

Work with the school and your child's teacher to provide sensory-motor breaks and/or physical activity. |

Figure 8.1. Supporting Healthy Habits in Children With Autism

Source: Derived from Curtin C, Hyman SL, Boas DD, et al. Weight management in primary care for children with autism: expert recommendations. *Pediatrics.* 2020;145(suppl 1):S126–S139.

Parents and caregivers of children on the autism spectrum are balancing many different needs and priorities, including different medical office visits, working with their child's school and therapists, and, sometimes, medications. In addition, they may be working on school avoidance, elopement, development of independent activities of daily living, or other situations. Striking a balance may require working on eating habits, expanding food preferences, and decreasing sedentary activity at a later time, or just making these needs a lower priority. Understandably, parents and caregivers may need to put this effort off. Some warning signs that food issues may need to be addressed sooner include weight changing dramatically (increasing or decreasing), a child eating items that aren't food (called *pica*), a child eating only 1 or 2 different items in each food group or avoiding entire food groups (ie, not eating any protein), food and mealtimes causing great anxiety or disruptive behavior, or a child showing no interest in food at all. If you and your family are experiencing any of these signs, talk with one of your medical providers, or have your child assessed by a dietitian or feeding specialist.

We have summarized the following 3 suggestions from what caregivers of children on the autism spectrum have told us over the years when they have concerns about eating habits:

- **Establish a routine.** You are likely already instituting some form of structure or routine to help your child learn and grow. Apply that routine to meals and snacks, physical activity, and electronics as you are able.
- **Changes may take twice as long.** Change is a slow process for any family, and for children on the autism spectrum, it can be even slower. Recognize that changes in eating and activity will take longer; allow time for your child to become familiar with a new food or change in routine first and ease them into it. Don't immediately ban electronics from dinnertime if that is part of their routine, as it could result in pushback. Try removing electronics at one meal, planning ahead to have other strategies (like a game) as a replacement initially. If your child doesn't make it through the entire meal without electronics, you've taken the first step. Don't give up if it takes weeks or months to get the new habit in place.

- **Take a deep breath.** Changes in eating and activity habits can be very difficult to make, and if your child has challenges with textures, picky eating, or communication, it makes changes even more difficult. This work takes patience. You are providing the environment for your child to slowly adjust eating behaviors. Pushing harder will backfire. Do your best without causing stress in yourself, your family, and your child.

> ### Picky Eating: My Sensory Experience
>
> "I've always been a picky eater. Some foods feel strange in my mouth, and certain smells make me want to gag. My dad has been encouraging me to try new foods for as long as I can remember. He says it's important, but it makes me feel anxious. I wish people understood that I'm not being difficult; it's just how my body reacts. Sometimes I get really upset when Dad doesn't make the foods I feel OK eating. I know if I push just enough, he'll give in and make my favorite (chicken nuggets and fries).
>
> But the other week, something felt different. He really made an effort to include foods I might actually eat. He asked me to join him for dinner instead of going to my room. I didn't want to at first, but when he said I could watch my phone while I ate, I thought maybe it wouldn't be so bad. I really prefer not to talk during meals—it helps me feel calm. That night, we had pasta with meat sauce. He also offered steamed broccoli and raw broccoli. He knows I gag on mushy textures, so I chose the raw broccoli. He let me make my plate, and I skipped the meat sauce and covered my noodles in Parmesan cheese. What surprised me most was that he didn't say anything about what was on my plate—no comments, no pressure. We just had a quiet, pleasant meal. I wish people knew that picky eating isn't about being stubborn. For me, it's about feeling safe and comfortable. And sometimes, that's really hard."
>
> —Alex, age 14

Attention-Deficit/Hyperactivity Disorder

A common stereotype of a child with attention-deficit/hyperactivity disorder (ADHD) is the child not wanting to eat because they take stimulant medication. Of course, it's more complex than that. Most studies have shown that children with ADHD actually have an overall increased risk for obesity. Why that is still confuses people but may have to do with dysregulated and erratic eating patterns coming from impulsivity. Other possible contributors linked to ADHD are more sedentary behaviors and electronics and screen time use. When ADHD is well managed, it can help lower that risk; while medications to treat ADHD will often lower a child's appetite during the day, they wear off at night and further dysregulate eating.

If your child has ADHD and is being treated, or your child is just starting the process of being diagnosed or treated for ADHD, do not stress about weight gain or, if medications are being used in the short term, don't panic about a small amount of weight loss (if you are unsure, check with your child's doctor to see if the amount of weight loss is worrisome). The use of structure, and not of pressuring or restricting, and doing it with warmth and love, will help you and your child through any challenges with activity or appetite. A daily and weekly schedule of meals and snacks, physical activity, and electronics time can easily incorporate medications or other behavioral approaches to treating ADHD. From our experience working with families and children with ADHD, the following approaches are very useful:

- **Plan ahead for the change.** Many ADHD medications can alter your child's appetite. The medications can lower the drive to eat or suppress hunger cues and can throw off children's typical eating patterns. Being ready for this effect and expecting it to happen will prevent the struggles and stress over food that can arise. Your child may bring home a half-eaten lunch or may report not eating much of the school lunch. It's OK; this was likely to happen, especially when the medication was first started. Your job is to roll with it and understand that the medications are influencing eating. You and your child are still doing your jobs well.

- **Don't push.** Pushing your child to eat when they aren't hungry is pressure, which we have seen to have negative repercussions. Avoid bribing or coaxing your child to eat during these times. Continue to offer meals and snacks on a schedule, being aware that their appetite has changed.
- **Modify the food schedule.** Work around the medications by keeping the meals on a schedule but making the following small changes:
  - Offering breakfast before medication is a chance to let hunger decide the amount eaten before the medication reduces your child's appetite. Having that meal before the medication starts working can really help.
  - Still offer or send lunch, but don't stress or turn it into a struggle to eat. If packing a lunch, ask them to help decide what goes into the lunch to ensure they are more likely to eat something. Or offer to pack a snack to take to lunch if they eat the school lunch. It's OK to send less food at lunch if they aren't finishing it, or let them know they can get something smaller from the cafeteria and not have to get a full lunch. No need to comment on the uneaten meal. Ellyn Satter's approach stresses that you did your job by providing it and trusting your child to decide how much to eat.
  - Offer a filling after-school snack as the medication wears off, or maybe switch to a bedtime snack if they aren't hungry after school. It is OK to build an eating schedule that provides more frequent late-day eating to accommodate when hunger increases.
  - Continue to let them eat as much or little as they choose at dinner. It may be more than you expect because they are catching up from the day.
  - Adding a bedtime snack is OK. If they are rummaging in the cabinets every night before bed, it is OK to add a scheduled snack time. Some nights they will want it, and other nights they may not. By adjusting the schedule, you are providing predictability for their eating. Their body is telling them to eat later in the day, and this is OK to allow but only at scheduled times.

- **Don't forget the Structure and Love approach.** This concept still holds true, especially in children with ADHD. Don't turn a lack of appetite into a struggle, and don't overindulge to get them to eat something. Even if they aren't very hungry, still have them sit down at the table or come to eat during mealtimes. While medications might dampen their hunger, sometimes the exposure to food will trigger another hunger pathway. Most important is keeping them on a routine and allowing them to listen to their bodies and hunger. Later in the evening, when medications have worn off, or there are less distractions at the meal (because you've slowly instituted the rule of no electronics at meals and snacks), they will hopefully sense their hunger and eat the food presented to them.

Much like with the parents of children on the autism spectrum, take pressure off yourself. For children with ADHD, you're trying to get them into a position to be successful in school and social settings. Addressing challenges head-on, by trying to make lots of changes in a short amount of time, will be very stressful and is likely to result in conflict in the home. Your first priority is getting your child's ADHD treated so they are doing well in school. Slowly instituting structure in meals and snacks, homework, and electronics-free time will help support that and hopefully lessen conflicts and relieve stress.

Medical Conditions to Consider

As we provide the environment to allow children to enjoy food and honor their hunger and fullness cues, we must also consider how to manage their medical exceptions. When the body's biology cannot tolerate a food, that food must be avoided. This can occur with illnesses such as food allergies or intolerances, gastrointestinal disorders such as Crohn disease or celiac disease, type 1 and 2 diabetes, irritable bowel syndrome, and others that restrict what foods our body can manage. The body must be respected, and these types of illnesses require adjustments to our children's intake. When gluten makes our body feel unwell, we avoid gluten. Here are some examples of how to modify a meal for specific medical conditions.

Chapter 8 | Picky Eating and Other Nutritional Challenges

"My child can't eat gluten, so I make a whole separate meal. How can we all eat together without making my child with a gluten allergy want the other foods?"

Offer a meal that has both regular and gluten-free options and that is similar. A family meal that considers the needs of family members would be chicken parmesan without breading, pasta and gluten-free pasta, and salad with croutons on the side.

"I have to sneak dessert to one child so my child with type 2 diabetes doesn't know we are having sweets. How do I handle this better?"

Begin by eating out in the open. When there is dessert, include a low-sugar option for all family members or similar regular and sugar-free options. Dessert could certainly be fruit with sugar-free whipped cream, or provide brownies made with a sugar substitute. Providing candy and similar sugar-free candy is another option. We do this not only to satisfy a need for sweet flavors but also to keep fairness among family members.

> Aminah's daughter has celiac disease and cannot eat gluten. Aminah cooks for her family of 5 and is frustrated with how to prepare a meal to meet the needs of her child with picky eating and be gluten-free. After meeting with a dietitian, she creates a list of meals that will work by making small accommodations in her meals. When she grills hamburgers, she has gluten-free buns for her daughter and has sides that her child with picky eating will enjoy. The key is that there is just one meal with a few variations for individual medical needs.

> David is not sure about how to cook meals now that his son has been diagnosed with an allergy to peanuts. This requires a lot of changes for safety. He is learning how to check labels for peanuts as an ingredient or whether the product was made in a nut-free manner. When he personally wants a meal that includes a peanut product, he knows he has to eat this away from home or when his son is at a friend's for the weekend. After much practice, he is feeling more confident with providing favorite meals but in a safe manner.

Treatment of some medical conditions includes medications that affect appetite. Appetite can decrease for part of the day, stay low all the time, or stay high all the time. When a medication overrides the body's message about hunger and fullness, our Structure and Love approach still applies. How do we do this? For structure, we continue to offer foods on a schedule. When appetite is high, keep on a schedule, and know your child will eventually adapt to this new way of eating. When appetite is low, continue with your schedule, and make sure that your child feels secure in their eating and that your love for them is felt. Allow satisfaction of hunger but only at the set eating times. Include foods that increase satiety, like protein and fiber. Remember that you can do this! Always consult a doctor if concerned about an eating disorder or if weight is declining rapidly.

Parental Eating Needs to Consider

For adults, there may also be reasons that foods are avoided or intake is adjusted. You may be making changes to eating because of bariatric surgery, low-sodium diets for high blood pressure, or medication for weight loss. Our advice here is simple: continue to provide meals on a schedule and eat together, with necessary additions so all family members have food to enjoy at the meal. What does this look like day-to-day? When a parent has a need for a low-sodium diet, everyone in the family can eat this way. All meals can avoid added salt. I know someone who grew up with a low-sodium diet for her parents. After the diagnosis of hypertension, meals stayed the same but cooking methods changed. Salt was replaced with other seasonings. Canned foods were replaced with the low-sodium type. Her parents ate everything without salt, but the children could add salt when needed. Meals were still delicious as the family adjusted to the new flavor options.

When taking weight loss medications or recovering from bariatric surgery, a parent may lose interest in preparing meals because of a decreased appetite. It is still the caregiver's role to provide a meal and stick with the schedule. When interest in cooking is low, recruit another family member to cook! One person can clean up if someone else does the cooking. You can also plan on ordering food in, trying quick meal options (premade or no cooking involved), or indulging in a meal kit delivery. I have said this before and I repeat it because even with medical or other reasons for adjusting parental eating, *the rest of the family still needs the meal provided.*

Parental avoidance of "bad" foods in the home affects family members by adding guilt or food preoccupation. When potato chips are not allowed in the home because a parent has an affinity for them, this may work well for the adult. It may also create a heightened focus on potato chips for the child, where it has become a forbidden fruit. When foods are not allowed because they are so desirable that we cannot trust ourselves with them, they can become even more appealing. The next time potato chips are available at a birthday party, a child may eat more than usual because the food has been forbidden and access is granted. If the food is "bad" because of a value the family holds (eg, animal products, which would be unacceptable for a vegan family), this is to be respected. If the food is "bad" because of fear of losing control when eating it, look to include it in moderation. We all need practice with the foods we love most. We have to learn to trust ourselves with these favorite foods, and that means we need them around. Most of the time, when we have a favorite food that we avoid buying, it's because we lose control with that food and don't trust ourselves with it. I recommend 2 things: change the label and grant permission. When a food is so delicious that you don't trust yourself with it, first relabel it. Rather than label it "bad" or "junk," call it by its name only (eg, *potato chips*) without judgment, or be honest and call it "delicious"! Second, in small amounts or periodically, start allowing the food in the home and practice eating it with permission to enjoy it. You may initially overeat as you adjust. When that happens, try again another week and see how the food is managed by the second, third, and fourth attempts. Completely forbidding a "bad" food makes it more desirable, while having it around will allow opportunities to practice trusting yourself with it. We try to find a balance between forbidding foods from being in the house altogether, which children may sense as restriction so their desire for it increases, and allowing these as special treats. Parents and caregivers should strive to set up a home food environment that makes eating in a balanced and healthy manner easier, yet not be so strict that no pleasurable, indulgent, or special-occasion foods are allowed. A simple example is birthday cake: a child should absolutely be able to enjoy cake or cupcakes on their birthday, or a slice of cake at their friend's birthday party, with the understanding that you aren't buying or baking a birthday cake every week.

When a Parent Takes a Medication That Affects Appetite

Whether related to weight loss efforts or illness, when a parent or caregiver is taking medication that affects their appetite, this can also have an impact on the family meal. It is possible that the adult's medication increases hunger or that their illness/condition and treatment decreases their hunger. As hunger is reduced, this can lead to reduced interest in planning meals, cooking, or even eating with the family.

Let's look at ways to balance parental appetite changes with family needs.

1. Prioritize what is most important to your family and what priorities are key for you: a predictable mealtime schedule, eating at the table, family meals, home-prepared meals, saving time, saving energy, maintaining routine, favorite foods, and safe foods, to name a few. Think through what you as a family want to prioritize and discuss it together as a family.
2. Write down the top 2 or 3 values during a Family Meeting.
3. For each value, write out what that could look like given all the family needs.
   a. This process may include asking each other questions such as "Is it most important to eat meals together no matter what the food?" "Is it most important to have meals prepared at home?" or "Can we adjust by having a takeout meal together at the table and meet some of our values?"
   b. For example, a family where someone has a peanut allergy will need to adjust what is in the kitchen and consider all foods brought into the home for safety. This can feel like a complete loss of favorite food items for others. The family can discuss not only the value of safety but also the value of other nutritious and tasty foods. The change could look like offering times where children can eat peanut products away from home or finding substitutions that are allergy-safe.
   c. Another example would be planning a Pizza and Movie Night. For whatever reason (eg, medical, surgical, allergy), this could pose a problem for a parent. Alternative plans can be made around that, such as substituting the pizza with takeout options or gluten-free pizza while still watching the movie, or consider going to the theater and ordering food from there.

> 4. Explore each idea and vote on your final plans as a team.
> 5. Remember to have grace for each other and work together considering the complexity of all needs and wants.

Mental Health Considerations

Nutrition can also be affected by our mental health. Mental health diagnoses may cause changes in eating behaviors related to seeking comfort, eating off schedule, or taking medications adjusting appetite. A mental health diagnosis of an eating disorder is in itself altered eating behavior. For all mental health impacts to nutrition, please consult with your child's pediatrician and/or mental health professional for guidance on your child's specific needs.

When mental health conditions such as anxiety or depression lead to eating for comfort, you may hear words like *emotional eating* or *comfort eating* being used to describe that type of behavior. You may feel that these are judgments and are wrong behaviors. We regularly hear caregivers describe their teenager as "an emotional eater." This description implies that emotional eating is wrong and must be corrected. I want to counter that judgment and allow the shift in mindset that food is comforting. It can be used as comfort. Certain emotions like anger, sadness, or worry can create physical feelings we think are hunger. Certain foods may help us feel better when we are upset, so it is important to recognize this behavior and not add guilt to it. We also need more than just one way to find comfort when we are upset. And there are still rules for when and where to eat. Help your child build a whole toolbox to manage their mood so eating is allowed as one of their options, but not the only option—where it can cause problems in the future. A therapist can be a huge help in building this toolbox. Sometimes when we are anxious, we eat a comforting meal. Other times when we are anxious, we can choose to write in a journal, call a friend to talk, listen to music, or play basketball. Comfort eating is encouraged to remain at scheduled times as much as possible. Removing guilt from this behavior is essential. Another common aspect of eating to soothe emotions is eating in private to hide the behavior. We want all eating behaviors to occur in the open. If eating for comfort is happening in the bedroom, one step to remove guilt can be to follow the rule of eating at the table. This transition gives permission for the eating as long as it is at the table and at a scheduled time. If you notice eating behaviors that concern you, especially loss of control with intake or eating significantly more food than would be expected, please consult your pediatrician or therapist for further evaluation. I want to affirm that eating for comfort is OK. Allowing permission to eat for comfort can ease guilt.

Some children are so narrow in their food preferences, it can affect them nutritionally, either as micronutrient/macronutrient deficiencies or poor growth. One mental health condition, avoidant/restrictive food intake disorder, or ARFID, is a newer condition and gaining awareness in the medical field. ARFID occurs when children's food preferences are so selective and narrow that their health becomes affected, slowing down their growth and development. Unlike other eating disorders, ARFID is not driven by weight concerns, body size, or appearance but arises from a complex set of factors such as neurodevelopmental differences (such as autism spectrum), psychological concerns (anxiety), or medical conditions (food allergies). Some children can have little interest in eating and seem to have very little hunger or have anxiety about particular foods. Sometimes this can occur because of a traumatic event such as choking on a food, after which they are scared to eat any food requiring chewing; because of sensitivity or a strong aversion to certain textures, smells, tastes, or appearances of food; or because of mental health conditions such as anxiety or obsessive-compulsive disorder. When a child is diagnosed with ARFID, occupational or speech therapy is recommended to assess feeding and to work with the child to increase comfort with food variety. A mental health professional is also recommended for this work when anxiety is part of the challenge. Just as with other eating disorders, nutritional impact can be dangerous, so professional support is essential. Maintain the same structure with eating, which supports predictability and shows parental patience for a slow change process. I recommend continuing to offer meals and snacks to your child and including foods they prefer so they always have a safe food at these eating times. Even if they do not eat all the foods offered, there is something they can safely fill up on at most eating times. Follow the picky eating guidance as a starting point (see the Picky Eating section earlier in this chapter), and add professional support to address nutritional concerns.

Health Concerns and Weight

The decision to pursue weight management for your child is an important one and best made as a family (depending on the age of your child) and your child's doctor. If you decide to do so, it's important to look for a program that specializes in child and adolescent health, involves working with families, follows expert guidelines and recommendations, and acknowledges the substantial time commitment. The path laid out in this book will still apply and support your family if attending a weight management program; also, we have covered things to watch out for in a program, such as actions that can risk disordered eating. Taking additional steps for your child to lose weight should be done carefully, and we encourage families to do so with a credible expert. Figure 8.2 is adapted from a *Journal of the Academy of Nutrition and Dietetics* article written by dietitians and researchers about safely caring for people with obesity while addressing weight stigma and eating disorder risk.

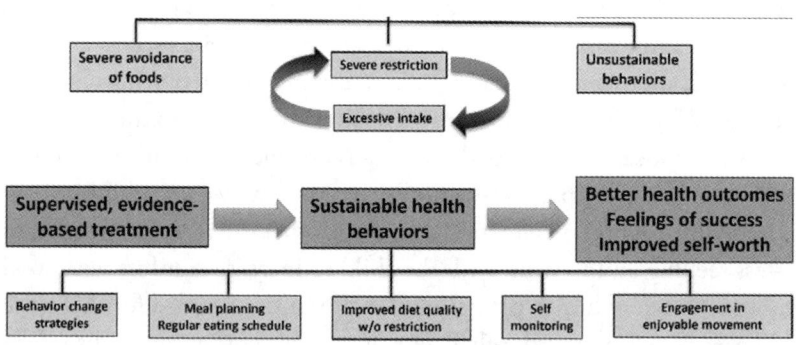

Figure 8.2. Dieting Versus Building Sustainable Health Behaviors

Source: Adapted from Cardel MI, Newsome FA, Pearl RL, et al. Patient-centered care for obesity: how health care providers can treat obesity while actively addressing weight stigma and eating disorder risk. *J Acad Nutr Diet.* 2022;122(6):1089–1098.

Chapter 8 | Picky Eating and Other Nutritional Challenges

While Figure 8.2 was created with adults in mind, it highlights some very important things:

- Trying to lose weight through diets or other ways that involve restricting what is eaten can be harmful, possibly increasing the risk for eating disorders and feelings of failure.
- Sustainable, lasting changes in our habits (learning how to change habits, meal planning, regular eating schedule, finding an activity that is enjoyable) will set your family up for success, even if there are not changes in weight.

What about Robin and Jaylen? One day, Robin decided she could no longer prepare 2 separate meals at dinner. It was just too much work and money. For a week or so, she still made Jaylen's favorite foods but served them right along with what she served the rest of the family, taking the focus off "his dinner" and instead making it a family dinner. She made sure there was at least one food he liked at each meal but did not make comments on him trying new foods or pressure him to eat. She also didn't pay attention to him when he ate only 1 or 2 items on his plate. Some nights she noticed that he ate only a few bites on his plate. She had to remind herself that he would be OK and would be able to eat again at his next mealtime. When he asked about more snacks later in the evening, she explained how the family was now eating on a schedule. He pushed back at first, but once they started being consistent with following the schedule, Robin noticed that Jaylen came to meals hungry and ready to eat the foods she cooked. If he was dissatisfied about dinner, she included him in planning meals for the week, which he loved. One day, he even asked if they could make a recipe he found online.

Chapter 9

You've Got This!

We want to raise healthy, happy children to be healthy, happy adults. This involves encouraging their education, developing a sense of right versus wrong, keeping them safe and healthy, and doing a million other things. As a pediatrician, I want children to be healthy now, as well as grow to be healthy adults, so they can feel good and do good. As a colleague once said, "We want to launch healthy kids into being healthy adults."

It's a Marathon, Not a Sprint

So focus on their health now but also keep an eye on the long term. For the longest time, people tried to be healthy by going on restrictive diets and doing punishing exercise routines to lose weight. We now know that this works only in the short term and will not lead to long-term weight loss and better health. In some cases, dieting strategies could be dangerous for people.

For a child in a bigger body, limiting how much they eat at meals, bribing them to exercise, and forbidding any fun foods could result in short-term weight loss but, over the long term, will damage their relationship with food, with their body, and with you...plus, these attempts at weight loss may result in even greater weight gain. Developing a lifetime approach to health and well-being can start in childhood, with your eye on the long-term impact. Short-term successes in changing nutrition, activity, and screen time habits are not achieving the goal of a lifetime of health and well-being. Changes you make as a parent, for you, your children, and your family, should be focused on the long term. You may not make a big change in your child's eating habits in the short term (maybe you still pack cheese puffs for lunch), but you do set them up for success in the long run by not causing harm to their self-esteem, building a positive body image, nurturing a healthy relationship with food (that includes eating cheese puffs without guilt), and incorporating positive family interactions about health instead of getting into constant battles.

Sustainable health habits without the negative side effects of dieting were highlighted by a group of nutrition researchers who proposed a framework for people wanting to manage their weight without harm, which they referred to as *sustainable health behaviors,* or, as I call them, "lifetime habits." We discussed their approach in Chapter 8, Picky Eating and Other Nutritional Challenges (see Figure 8.2). We now translate those sustainable health behaviors for families, as found in this book:

- Applying parenting strategies to change family habits (authoritative parenting, or the Structure and Love approach; see Chapter 2.)
- Lowering pressure and restriction (See Chapter 2.)
- Implementing family schedules: using family meetings, posting schedules for the family to see (See Chapter 2.)
- Spending time together: communicating well; doing more activities together, from playing games to preparing meals (See Chapters 3, 4, and 5.)
- Practicing meal planning and regular eating schedules (See Chapter 6.)
- Applying parenting approaches to being active as a family (See Chapter 7.)
- Approaching picky eating and other challenges (See Chapter 8.)

Raising Healthy Children in an Unhealthy World

When you think about wanting the best for your children, it's easy to get caught up in the short-term, or immediate, challenges in front of you, such as

- Your child is being teased about their weight.
- Their cholesterol level is rising.
- Type 2 diabetes runs in the family, and your child's blood glucose (sugar) level is starting to rise.

- Your child is on screens all the time and getting little to no exercise.

Every parent and caregiver would want to do something to help their children. At the same time, there are long-term goals when it comes to their health and well-being: preventing chronic disease, as well as promoting high self-esteem and positive body image, a healthy relationship with food, and strong family connections.

When you are making changes to your child and family health habits, remember that there are potential harms that can come from addressing those habits, ranging from disordered eating to damaged self-esteem to stress on the family. Your child may not get to a weight that is considered healthy by the standards of a growth chart, either now in their childhood or later as an adult. Compare that against the stress and potential damage that can come from focusing too much on diet and exercise: low self-esteem and negative body image and a lifelong focus on weight. Thousands of body positivity activists have shared heart-wrenching stories of pain, broken relationships, and disordered eating that arose from efforts to be a certain size, including negative and hurtful interactions from people who were trying to be helpful. The potential harm that can come from focusing too much on short-term improvements in diet, activity levels, and weight can be undone by the long-term side effects. Many parents have relayed to us over the years how they don't want their children to grow up disliking their bodies, being too preoccupied with calories and minutes of vigorous physical activity, being too obsessed with their weight, and basing their self-esteem and feelings of self-worth on how their body looks. These parents come to us because they want to find a different way to raise their children to be healthy in an unhealthy world, one with kindness, family closeness, and, yes, you guessed it, love.

The Structure and Love approach allows us to put guardrails on the world around us. It takes practice, and the stories and guidance provided in this book can give you a game plan. No one will be perfect, and know you can't do it alone. Look for support from your spouse/partner. Some social science researchers look at families through a lens of flexibility and cohesion through what is called the Circumplex Model of Marital and Family Systems, which I further detail in the following lists. It kind of reminds me of the story of Goldilocks and the 3 bears, where the porridge on either side is too hot or too cold, but the porridge in the middle is just right.

Flexibility, or adaptability: How structured, organized, or "go with the flow" is your family?

- If families are too *rigid,* they struggle to make changes. If crises occur that require change, the family struggles even more to adapt or overcome the crises and can suffer.
- If families are too *flexible,* the home and family can become chaotic. A lack of structure makes it difficult to make a change in schedule or habits, much less to be organized enough to overcome a crisis.

Cohesion: How close or separated are family members?

- If families are too close, or *enmeshed,* people can lose a sense of their own individuality, struggle to become their own person, and never benefit from having privacy.
- If families are too separated, or *disengaged,* they don't form strong feelings of attachment, belonging, and security in their family. This lack of connection can interfere with people's ability to develop close relationships later in life.

Aim for "in the middle": have rules and structure but enough flexibility to allow for growth, change, and spontaneity. Have closeness and strong relationships but some independence to allow for individuality and personal space. The key to this is *communication*! Positive communication, whether that is talking, spending time together, or staying in contact, can help keep families in that happy middle ground. Balance is navigating between extremes and finding that sweet spot, in the middle, for your family.

Let's Review

As you prepare to make changes at home, let's take a quick look back at where we've been together and what the Structure and Love Approach involves. To build self-esteem, remove food preoccupation and sneaking, and encourage balance with eating and activities, we recommend these shifts. Although they are simple on the surface, we believe in them wholeheartedly. Research shows that implementing these recommendations can make a huge difference in the how of eating and moving as a family.

- **Involve the entire family in making habit shifts together.** Your family team, whatever the size of your crew, needs to have input so they are invested in the plans. Your family is your greatest strength. Importantly, changes made to support a child with weight concerns should apply to all siblings living in the home, even if they don't share the same challenges. This approach helps prevent any child from feeling singled out and encourages full participation. Working together will make the effort as successful as possible. Capitalize on teamwork, hearing everyone's voices, in all ways that you can as you get started.
- **Create a routine and practice consistency to establish your structure.** Take into consideration your household's typical week, including set times to eat meals and snacks, and your household's evening commitments and bedtimes. Since communication is key, get your team's input and then post this schedule for all to see. Consider sharing the weekly schedule by text or posting it in multiple locations, whichever is best for clear communication in your home.
- **Plan ahead for meals and snacks to make food available for your family.** As caregivers, you are in charge of providing the food for both meals and snacks, whether that is at home or from a restaurant. Planning in advance (1–2 days in advance or a full week) helps you purchase groceries and have options ready when it is time to eat. Remember, you won't be labeling foods as "healthy" or "unhealthy" and you won't have to get in the weeds of what you "should" be eating. Indulgent foods are allowed and provided as you decide for them to be provided.
- **Remember the P & R Coin.** Pressure and restriction can lead to stress for you and your child. Your job with meals and snacks is done once you've provided the food options. Let your child take it from there. Be mindful of your words and body language. No need to push them to eat more vegetables or stop them from getting a second helping. It will only backfire. Every family hopes for mealtimes to be happy, pleasant experiences.

By focusing on topics other than food at the table, you and your child can reduce stress and strengthen family connections.
- **Model behaviors you want to see in your children to show rather than just tell them what to do.** When you provide structure, your children and teens have the environment to follow the family habit changes well. Modeling takes this to another level and lets them see what to do as well. Modeling can involve showing kindness in your words about bodies and weight. Modeling can also involve removing pressure and restriction when talking about food and activity. Remove comments about whether the food is good or bad or what amount has been eaten. Once the meal is ready, sit back, relax, and enjoy your time together in a stress-free eating environment for everyone.
- **Make time to connect over meals.** As a reminder, we recommend eating as many family meals together as possible with electronics off. You can also adapt this recommendation for your household's schedules and needs. When time allows for a family meal together, encourage conversation to connect. Show love by showing interest in topics that interest the rest of the family, by sharing part of your day or your experiences with the others at the meal.
- **Schedule activities together, which is the most fun part of all.** As a family, take time to identify what kinds of activities work for individuals and for the group. Listen to everyone's preferences, and arrange time to have fun. Whether your family takes an after-dinner walk together, has a dance party in the kitchen, or plays a new card game, you are practicing a new habit together. Whether it is physical activity or screen-free activity (like the card game), your family is creating new habits together and possibly even family traditions.

The Structure and Love approach provides the basic support that growing children and teens need. From the parenting model discussed in Chapter 2, Parenting Through Structure and Love, the how of parenting with an authoritative approach includes these key concepts. You, as the expert on your family, get to decide which pieces you want to implement in your home. You, as the expert on your family, get to decide how often the new habits can happen. And the more you practice, the more you build consistency and make lasting changes for all.

"This approach still seems a little weird to me."

Yes, we understand. This approach of staying away from pressure or restriction, avoiding body and weight talk, creating schedules, and allowing indulgent foods goes against the prevailing sentiment of "helping" children make changes by guiding them to live the lives you want of them or even controlling the amounts they eat and the time they spend on screens. We want to *fix* things! (They weigh too much? Cut back on what they are eating and make them move more.) What we have presented is based on science—the science of parenting, feeding dynamics, child development, and the family. The past 30 years of the "war on obesity" (public health efforts focused mainly on reducing excess weight) hasn't had many victories. While a lot of what we have covered in this book is known, there is much that hasn't been included in child and teen weight management programs and especially hasn't made it into popular culture (much less social media). For nearly 20 years, we've been learning in our program how to "thread the needle" of helping children be happy and healthy.

The rising rate of eating disorders in children in bigger bodies has only recently been recognized. We've known for years that there is a risk for eating disorders in this world of diet and exercise but thought it was limited to children who had underweight or looked a certain way, but we now know that's not the case. Knowing the risk for disordered eating in children should guide how we parent children around food and physical activity.

Year after year, scientists have really come to understand the complexity of our body size and weight. Some of it has been known for quite a while: our nutrition and activity habits, our genetic makeup, and our environment. More is known every year, especially around the science of how our body fights to stay the same weight. And there is still more we either don't know or are just learning about, such as endocrine-disrupting chemicals, ultra-processed foods, environmental changes, racism, weight bias, and epigenetics. We don't know all the contributors to our body size, so we should consider this complexity when we are trying to figure out the answers to "Why am I gaining weight?" or "Why are my children different sizes?"

As with many things in life, we have to remember the witticism that insanity is doing the same thing over and over and expecting a different result. We've not sufficiently recognized that trying to put our children on diets, or tricking them into being active, will not do anything substantial for them. We've been pressuring or restricting our children when we know this approach won't help, and it could possibly harm them. We know the risks for, at best, a damaged self-esteem and, at worse, eating disorders while not fully repudiating weight talk, restrictive diets, and weight teasing and bias. We've also realized that the public perceptions of beauty, and now health, are not realistic and set children and adults up to dislike their own bodies. Unfortunately, we still live in that world. While there are positive movements and changes going on (body positivity, models reflecting a variety of body sizes and types, and scientifically based approaches to health), our prevailing culture still has an idealized body type, making a number of people willing to sell you a quick fix that is not based on reputable science.

We use the themes of "Cook, Eat, Play, Repeat" to put these complex ideas into our daily lives. In the following table of those themes, we have goals on the left side and reasons why these goals are important on the right:

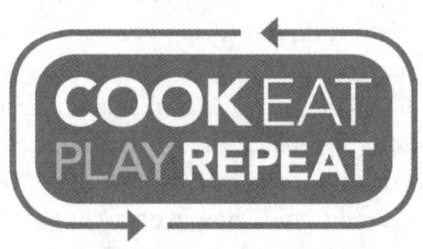

COOK at home	
✓ Eat most meals at home ✓ Plan meals ahead of time ✓ Make foods your family likes ✓ Cook one meal for everyone	Aim to cook and eat at home most of the time. This will save you time and money and add more variety to your meals.
	Create a meal plan in advance and decide when you will do your grocery shopping.
	Cook meals that your family enjoys and that feel special to you. Eating familiar foods makes mealtime more fun.
	Prepare one meal that the whole family can enjoy. If children get used to having separate meals, they may never learn to like the foods you prepare.

EAT together

✓ Have 4 or more family meals each week ✓ Set a schedule for eating ✓ Turn off electronics while eating ✓ Remove pressure and restriction around eating	Research shows that family meals are important, as they help families communicate better and provide many benefits for children.
	Children and adults eat better when meals and snacks happen at regular times. Aim for 3 meals and 1 or 2 snacks each day.
	Using electronics and being distracted during meals can make it harder to recognize when you're hungry or full. Try turning them off during meals and snacks.
	When children are trusted to choose how much to eat, they become better at managing their hunger and eating the right amount for their bodies.

PLAY often

✓ Find activities your child/teen enjoys ✓ Model being active ✓ Schedule family playtime/physical activity ✓ Remove pressure and restriction around family play and physical activities	Brainstorm fun activities to do together, considering your child's likes and dislikes.
	When kids see you being active, they'll want to join in. Show them it's fun by trying new things together as a family!
	Whether it's a walk after dinner, a weekend bike ride, or a game of soccer in the yard, setting aside time for activities like these shows your children that staying active is important.
	Provide opportunities for your child to participate and let them choose how much they want to engage—whether it is a lot or a little. Removing pressure helps them feel in control and more open to being active.

REPEAT	
✓ Make cooking, eating, and playing a routine ✓ Get the whole family involved ✓ Practice new habits one at a time ✓ Create a routine for bedtime	Doing these activities regularly helps your family bond and develop healthy habits.
	Working together builds teamwork and makes it easier to change habits successfully.
	To make changes easier, start with a small change, and once that feels comfortable, gradually add another habit.
	A consistent sleep schedule can improve your child's health, boost their mood, and help them focus better during the day.

Advocate for You and Your Child

As you moved through this book and began to understand this complexity, you probably realized that most people don't understand how complex body size is, how conventional approaches to changing habits can actually cause harm, and that children are different from adults. Undoubtedly, no matter what your child's body type, you will get advice from people on parenting, whether you asked for it or not. Remember that this usually comes from a good place, wanting to help (although we all have that friend or family member who should keep their advice to themselves!). Sometimes this advice is being shared in front of your child, or the person may try to institute a new habit for your child in your place. Frustrating for sure! Sometimes people in positions of authority or importance in you and your child's life even try to "help," and it may be the opposite of help, such as

- Commenting on your child's weight because they want to "make you aware"
- Offering nutrition or exercise advice to "keep your child healthy"
- Suggesting adult-focused health programs for your child
- Trying to motivate your child by saying how great they will look if they "lose a few pounds"

If you sense someone is trying to "help," gently put a stop to it. Sometimes it can be as simple as saying, "Other people's bodies are none of our business," or calling attention to how certain things can be harmful in children, like calorie counting or frequent weighing. It's also an opportunity to educate, sharing how dieting, weight talk, teasing, and shaming someone's body can lead to eating disorders. As we talked about in Chapter 3, (Not) Talking With Your Kids About Their Weight, when it comes to bullying, use your best judgment on how thoroughly you want to discuss the topic with someone. It's enough to say, "Body size is very complicated, because it's not just nutrition and exercise. Let's not get into that right now." I very commonly speak with caregivers in the clinic alone, so children don't misinterpret what is meant when weight is discussed. Take that approach if someone says something to your child: "It's complicated. Let's talk about it later." Depending on the situation, feel inspired to take it a step further: "Talking about weight with children can be very damaging." In the end, you might even just say, "We're on top of it." Take the opportunity to share resources like this book and others that can support children, and families, to be healthy *and* happy.

Just like with friends and family, many health care professionals don't understand the full complexity of body weight, and they carry some of the same harmful "diet and exercise" ideas the rest of the world does. Unfortunately, weight bias within health professions is well documented. Hopefully, your family will not encounter this bias, but if you do, continue to advocate and protect your children. Many size acceptance groups encourage individuals to request not to be weighed or not to discuss weight unless necessary to deliver safe and effective care, such as having to calculate the correct dose of a medication based on a person's weight. If your child's health care professional makes a comment about weight that could or does upset your child, ask to speak with them privately, and share your feelings. Using some of the same tips we've provided in this book, note that you are aware of your child's weight and are addressing it in a way that is safe and not upsetting to your child. Request that they not address issues about weight (unless that is something you and your child want to discuss with them), and keep the discussion focused on habits that impact health, not weight. If this is something you have encountered before, or you are changing health care professionals as a result, bring it up at the first visit.

The Beatles summarized what we are saying about families quite well in a song: all you need is love! We know it's not that simple, but it is the foundation of a family, the core of being a parent, and our touchstone as we navigate making changes in our family. Being a newly crowned empty nester, I can tell you that love does not stop when teenagers leave the house. The love for my 2 boys, my wife, and my family as a whole only grows stronger the older, and hopefully wiser, I get. Every year, I recognize how important that love is and how to relay that love to my children so they know it. Showing interest in them, who they are and the person they want to be; listening to them; and just simply spending time with them—these are what let your children know you love them.

Let's Get Started!

It's time to change the narrative! This book has given you the tools to understand how to make small changes that can have a big impact, not just for your child but for your whole family. Yes, what we eat matters for our health. But today, there's so much messaging and confusion around food that it's hard to know what's truly right or wrong. If you lead your family through these changes by focusing on **how** you eat, rather than stressing over **what** you eat, you'll help your child build a healthy relationship with food that lasts a lifetime. This approach can protect them from getting pulled into the world of dieting as they grow. There will be bumps along the way, and that's OK. Start slowly. Make changes together as a family. And remember: every step sets your child up for success.

Appendix

Throughout this book, we have referenced various activity-based figures or tables. In the following pages, you will find those figures or tables from each chapter turned into templates for your own individual use. We encourage you to use these general templates with your family. They fall into themes we call "Cook, Eat, Play, Repeat," introduced in Chapter 9, You've Got This!, as part of the Structure and Love approach and meant to support your family in establishing health habits around eating and physical activity.

Eating and Activity Habits Survey

Use this survey to assess where your family is with important habits that will make a big impact on the health of your child and family.

Check one box for each statement.

COOK at home

1. We eat most of our meals at home.
   ☐ Almost always   ☐ Often   ☐ Sometimes   ☐ Almost never

2. We plan meals ahead of time.
   ☐ Almost always   ☐ Often   ☐ Sometimes   ☐ Almost never

3. We cook meals that our family enjoys and that feel special.
   ☐ Almost always   ☐ Often   ☐ Sometimes   ☐ Almost never

4. We prepare one meal for everyone in the family.
   ☐ Almost always   ☐ Often   ☐ Sometimes   ☐ Almost never

EAT together

5. We have 4 or more family meals together each week.
   ☐ Almost always   ☐ Often   ☐ Sometimes   ☐ Almost never

6. We follow a regular schedule for meals and snacks (3 meals and 1–2 snacks each day).
   ☐ Almost always   ☐ Often   ☐ Sometimes   ☐ Almost never

7. We turn off electronics during meals and snacks.
   ☐ Almost always   ☐ Often   ☐ Sometimes   ☐ Almost never

8. We practice removing pressure and restriction around eating.
   ☐ Almost always   ☐ Often   ☐ Sometimes   ☐ Almost never

PLAY often

9. We find activities our child/teen enjoys doing.
   ☐ Almost always   ☐ Often   ☐ Sometimes   ☐ Almost never

10. We model being active.
    ☐ Almost always   ☐ Often   ☐ Sometimes   ☐ Almost never

11. We schedule time for family play or physical activities.
    ☐ Almost always   ☐ Often   ☐ Sometimes   ☐ Almost never

12. We practice removing pressure and restriction around family play and physical activities.
    ☐ Almost always   ☐ Often   ☐ Sometimes   ☐ Almost never

Appendix

REPEAT

13. We make cooking, eating, and playing part of our regular routine.
    ☐ Almost always   ☐ Often   ☐ Sometimes   ☐ Almost never

14. Our whole family gets involved in making habit changes to improve our health.
    ☐ Almost always   ☐ Often   ☐ Sometimes   ☐ Almost never

15. We practice new habits one at a time to make changes easier.
    ☐ Almost always   ☐ Often   ☐ Sometimes   ☐ Almost never

16. We follow a consistent bedtime routine for our child.
    ☐ Almost always   ☐ Often   ☐ Sometimes   ☐ Almost never

Now review your responses.

Items marked as happening *sometimes* or *almost never* are areas where your family might choose to set new goals.

Depending on your survey responses, use the following information to help your family make changes:

COOK at home

The key to cooking and eating more meals at home, to ensuring that one meal is provided for the whole family, and to having meals that your family enjoys and that feel special is to plan ahead. Meal planning helps set the stage for success and allows for fine-tuning of routines that support better eating habits.

Appendix

The At-Home Meal Playbook (Chapter 6)

Getting Started:

- **Step 1**: Write down a list of Meals to Remember
- **Step 2**: Create a meal plan for the upcoming week
- **Step 3**: Make a grocery list
- **Step 4**: Plan a day to do your grocery shopping
- **Step 5**: Follow through with your plan

Meals to Remember Template (Chapter 6)

Meals to Remember

Entrées	Sides

Appendix

Meal Theme Nights Template (Chapter 6)

Sunday:	Monday:	Tuesday:	Wednesday:	Thursday:	Friday:	Saturday:

Weekly Family Meal Plan (Chapter 6)

Sunday	Monday	Tuesday	Wednesday	Thursday	Friday	Saturday

Evening Activities

Who's Cooking?

EAT together

Research shows that family meals are important because they help families communicate better and offer many benefits for children. Taking time to disconnect from electronics during meals also supports this connection and encourages everyone to eat more mindfully, paying closer attention to hunger and fullness cues. By allowing your child to stop eating when they feel full and satisfied with the meal that is offered, you're showing you trust them to listen to their own body. We find that shifting the focus away from the food and toward connection can have a big impact. Here are some questions and statements that can help get the conversation flowing.

Mealtime Conversation Starters

Get the conversation flowing at dinner by taking turns answering the following questions or statements. (For more ways on how to have a successful meal, see Chapter 6, specifically the Making Family Meals Happen section.)

What do you want to be when you grow up?	If you could be an animal, what would you be and why?	What is your favorite place in the whole world and why?
What superpower would you like to have?	If you had to leave the Earth on a spaceship, what 3 things would you take with you?	If you could eat dinner with someone famous, whom would you pick?
Share something nice that someone did for you today!	If you could be any type of food, what would you be and why?	What has been your favorite part about today? Why?
If you were to write a book about yourself, what would the title be?	Describe something you would like your family to do together in the future.	Finish this sentence: If I won a million dollars, I would _____.

Describe your perfect day, from the time you wake up...until the time you fall asleep!	If you could ride any animal, which would you choose?	What is your ultimate vacation?
Spring, summer, fall, or winter? Which is your favorite season and why?	Name 3 things you can't live without.	If you were a cereal, what kind would you be and why?

Meal Schedule

Children and adults eat better when meals and snacks happen at regular times. Aim for 3 meals and 1 to 2 snacks each day. Writing the schedule down and posting it in the home where everyone can see it can help the whole family follow it more consistently.

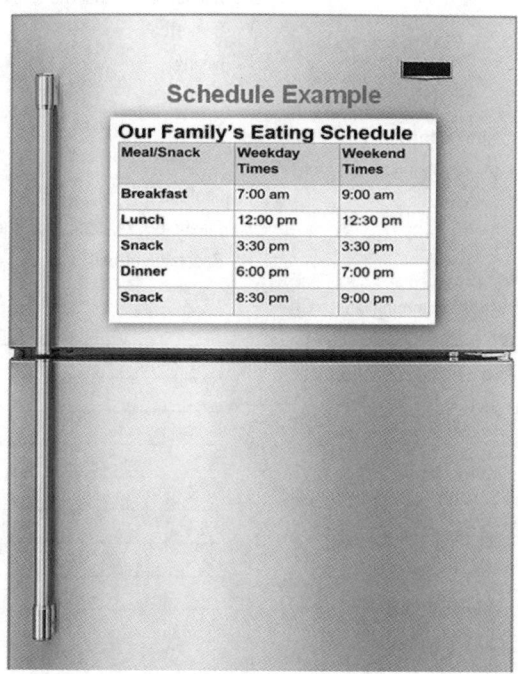

Schedule Example

Our Family's Eating Schedule

Meal/Snack	Weekday Times	Weekend Times
Breakfast	7:00 am	9:00 am
Lunch	12:00 pm	12:30 pm
Snack	3:30 pm	3:30 pm
Dinner	6:00 pm	7:00 pm
Snack	8:30 pm	9:00 pm

Appendix

PLAY often

Helping your child or teen stay active starts with finding activities they enjoy. Take time to brainstorm fun things to do together based on their interests. When children see you being active, they're more likely to join in, especially if it looks fun! Scheduling regular family activity time, like a walk after dinner or a weekend bike ride, shows that staying active is a priority. It's also important to practice removing the pressure to be active, as that often backfires, reducing activity. Giving them the freedom to choose helps them feel more in control and open to being active.

Family Activity Ideas (Chapter 7)

Place a check mark next to the activities your family enjoys. Add your own ideas in the blank spaces.

- ☐ Weight lifting, strength training
- ☐ Martial arts
- ☐ Gymnastics
- ☐ Running
- ☐ Dancing
- ☐ Twirling a hoop around the waist
- ☐ Walking in the neighborhood or at a park
- ☐ Tag
- ☐ Relay race
- ☐ Obstacle course
- ☐ Playing in the water, swimming laps
- ☐ Arts and crafts
- ☐ Games such as chase, tag, or hopscotch
- ☐ Using a jump rope
- ☐ Board games
- ☐ Playing on a playground
- ☐ Riding bikes
- ☐ Skateboarding, skating, rollerblading
- ☐ Volleyball
- ☐ Outdoor play, climbing trees, hide-and-seek

- ☐ Soccer
- ☐ Racket sports: badminton, tennis, pickleball
- ☐ Basketball
- ☐ Hiking
- ☐ Bowling
- ☐ Yoga
- ☐ 4 square
- ☐ Football
- ☐ Plastic bricks, cars, and other active toys
- ☐ Baseball/softball
- ☐ _____
- ☐ _____
- ☐ _____
- ☐ _____
- ☐ _____
- ☐ _____
- ☐ _____
- ☐ _____
- ☐ _____
- ☐ _____

Overlapping Family Activities (Chapter 7)

Make a list of activities you want to try, and have your child fill their circle out as well. Place the mutual activities into the middle of the diagram.

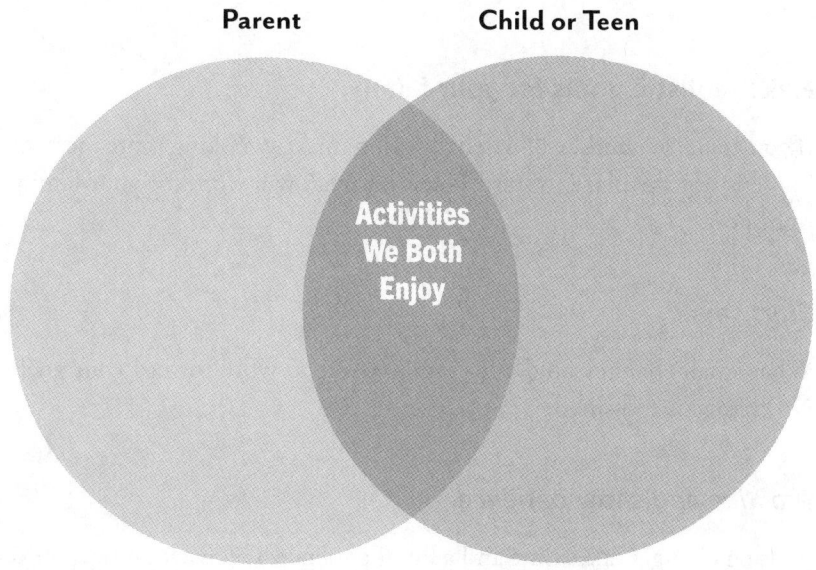

Appendix

REPEAT

Keep the following tips in mind when it comes to cooking at home, eating together, and playing often:

Make realistic goals for your family.

If you are in the middle of baseball season, maybe cooking more meals at home is not the place to start. Focus on what will work for your family right now.

Start small.

What small change could your family make to work toward your goal? No change is too small.

Practice and show patience.

Making changes takes time and a lot of patience. Get back on track next week if this week does not go as planned.

Celebrate successes.

Encourage each other when you make even the smallest step forward. You are in this together, and motivating each other is the key to making changes as a family.

Here are examples of family goals.

- Eat dinner together at the table twice a week.
- Follow our family eating schedule.
- Eat dinner together without the distraction of screens.
- Focus on my family at mealtimes and not on what my child is or isn't eating.

Appendix

The Importance of Sleep

A consistent sleep schedule can improve your child's health, boost their mood, and help them focus better during the day. (For more on what this schedule looks like, see Chapter 2, specifically the "Does this apply to sleep too?" box.)

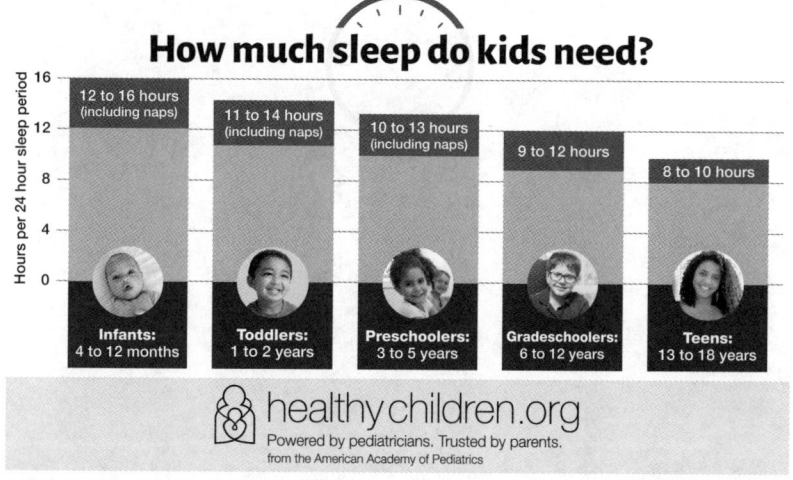

*The American Academy of Pediatrics (AAP) has issued a Statement of Endorsement supporting these guidelines from the American Academy of Sleep Medicine (AASM).

Source: Paruthi S, Brooks LJ, D'Ambrosio C, Hall W, Kotagal S, Lloyd RM, Malow B, Maski K, Nichols C, Quan SF, Rosen CL, Troester MM, Wise MS. Recommended Amount of Sleep for Pediatric Populations: A Statement of the American Academy of Sleep Medicine. *J Clin Sleep Med.* 2016 May 25. pii: jc-00158016. PubMed PMID: 27250809.

Index

Page numbers followed by *f* indicate a figure; by *t*, a table.

A
Active video games, 145
Adaptive exercise specialists, 144
Adipose tissue, 11, 12, 63
Advocating for children, 198–200
Affirmation of children's bodies, 23–25
Air pollution, 16
Allergies, 144
    food, 161*t*
Allostatic load, 12
American Academy of Pediatrics (AAP), 4, 14
    on eating disorders, 19
    Family Media Plan, 151
    on healthy media habits, 139–140
American Medical Association, 14
Anorexia nervosa, 161*t*
Anxiety, 161*t*
Asthma, 144
At-home meal playbook. *See* Planning, meal
Attention-deficit/hyperactivity disorder (ADHD), 161*t*, 176–178
Authoritative parenting, 136

Autism spectrum, 161*t*, 171–175, 173*f*
Avoidant/restrictive food intake disorder, 22, 161*t*, 185

B
Bariatric surgery, 75, 80, 84–85
Baumrind, Diana, 34
Bias, 12, 71, 196, 199
Binge-eating disorder, 161*t*
Birch, Leann, 40
Blended families, 95
Body mass index (BMI), 13–14
Body size and shape
    affirmation of children's, 23–25
    breaking generational myths about, 87
    metabolically healthy obesity and, 27–28
    positive reinforcement and, 25–29
    recognizing and honoring familial differences in, 79–80
    science behind, 13–17
    variance in, 12

Index

Body talk, positive, 26, 61–62
Bowen, Murray, 91
Brenner FIT (Families in Training) program, 5
Bribing with picky eating, avoiding, 170
Budgets, food, 114–115
Bullying and teasing, 67–72

C

"Calories in, calories out" myth, 13
Cancer, as related to allostatic load, 12
Celiac disease, 161*t*, 178
Center of Excellence on Social Media and Youth Mental Health, 139
Children
   advocating for, 198–200
   affirming the bodies of, 23–25
   age guidelines for healthy habits in, 38
   learning to trust, 168–169
   maturity level of, 37
   raised in an unhealthy world, 190–192
   reactions and behavior of, 36–37
   research on diets of, 41–42
   at risk for eating disorders, 21
   sleep needs of, 211
   uniqueness of, 37–38
Chronic disease, 12
Circumplex Model of Marital and Family Systems, 191
Cohesion, family, 192
Comfort eating, 184
Communication, family, 92–93, 98–99, 192
Comparison, avoiding, 25, 79
Conversations, 64–65
   addressing necessary, 65
   addressing teasing and bullying, 67–72
   avoiding comparison in, 25, 79
   avoiding talking about weight, 61–62
   about bariatric surgery, 84–85
   being honest in, 78
   considering choice of words used in, 65–66
   discussing what has happened since they made a habit change, parents, 80–82
   during family meals, 128–129, 206–207
   in family meetings, 58–60
   hidden meanings of the word *health* in, 63–64
   keeping things positive and within reason, 78–79
   meaning and impact of words in, 64–66
   parents talking about their own health with children, 78–85
   recognizing and honoring familial differences in bodies, 79–80
   about weight loss medications, 83–84
   what to focus on in, 66–67

Cooking at home, 108–111, 196, 203–205
Crohn disease, 161*t*, 178
Cycle of pressure, 129, 130*f*

D
Davis, Clara, 41–42
Deception with picky eaters, avoiding, 170–171
Depression, 161*t*
Diabetes, 12, 144, 161*t*, 178
Discrimination, 12
Disengaged, families too, 192
Disordered eating, 22–23
Divorce, blended families parenting around food after, 95

E
Eating behavior, 160
    mental health and, 161*t*, 184–187
    parental eating needs and, 161*t*, 181–184
    picky eating. *See* Picky eating
Eating disorders, 19, 20
    children at risk for, 21
    differences between disordered eating and, 22–23
Eating habits, 10
    at-home meal playbook and, 111–123
    and changing the family structure for the better, 85–86
    cooking at home, 108–111, 196, 203–205
    differences between children's and adults', 82–83
    disordered, 22–23
    family meals, 47–51, 100, 123–124, 127–132, 166, 194, 197, 206–207
    healthy relationship with food and, 126
    ingredient households versus snack households, 125–126
    modeling and, 58
    repeated exposure and, 57–58
    schedules and, 104–108, 165, 193
    survey on, 201–203
Eating in the absence of hunger, 107
Electronics use
    caregivers and children at odds over, 148–149
    during family meals, 128
    how to avoid disagreements over, 149–151
    preventing physical activity, 138–139
    shaping behavior with, 151–152
Emotional eating, 161*t*, 184
Enmeshed, families too, 192
Environmental factors in weight, 16–17
Exercise. *See* Physical activity
Exercise videos, 145

F

Families
  busy schedules of, 137–138
  cohesion of, 192
  communication within, 92–93, 98–99, 192
  connections in, 90–93
  eating meals together, 47–51, 100, 123–124, 127–132
  family meetings and, 58–60, 157
  grandparents in, 96–97
  influence on children's habits, 20
  making changes as, 98–99
  positive structure changes in, 85–86
  sabotage in, 94–95
  on the same team, 94–96
  spending time together, 99
  teamwork within, 100–101
  uniqueness of, 93–94
  See also Parenting
Family meals, 47–51, 100, 123–124, 127–132, 194, 197, 206–207
  diving into conversation during, 128–132
  picky eating and, 166
  putting ideas into action, 132
  tips for more, 127–128
  turning off electronics during, 128
Family therapy, 101
Fat, what is meant by "extra weight," 11
Fat, use of word, 27, 64–66

Fat Talk, 63
First Bite: How We Learn to Eat, 163
First-order change, 92
Food, access to, 16
Food neophobia, 164, 167
Food preferences, 163
Food regression, 163
Frozen food, 115–116

G

Gardening, 145
Gaslighting, affirming in place of, 24–25
Gastrointestinal disorders, 161*t*
Generational myths, 87
Genetics and weight, 16
Gluten-free diets, 161*t*
Grandparents, 96–97
Grocery shopping, 109–110, 116

H

Health, meaning of word, 63–64
Health Psychology, 54
Healthy, reframing the concept of, 26–27, 54–60
  avoiding labeling foods and, 56–58
  defining what healthy means and, 55–56
Healthy habits, 6–7, 11, 16–17
  family influence on, 20–21
  guidelines by age, 38
  helping children (safely) build, 19–21

as a marathon, not a sprint, 189–190
parenting around, 36–38
positive reinforcement of, 25–29
realistic goals for, 210
sustainable, 190
in an unhealthy world, 190–192
Healthy relationship with food, 126
Heart disease, 12
High blood pressure, 12
Hiking, 145
Hunger, 107–108

I
Indoor activities, budget-friendly, 145–146
Inflammation, 12, 144
Ingredient households versus snack households, 125–126
International Journal of Behavioral Nutrition and Physical Activity, 7
International Journal of Obesity, 64
Intuitive eating, 128
Irritable bowel syndrome, 161*t*, 178

J
Journal of Health, Population and Nutrition, 16

Journal of the Academy of Nutrition and Dietetics, 186
"Junk foods," 55

K
Keto diets, 161*t*

L
Labeling of foods, 56–58
Leftovers, 114, 122
Love
applied to activity, 46
applied to appetite, 47–49
applied to sleep, 45
expression of, 25, 34
in Structure and Love approach, 31, 36, 42–43, 136, 178, 180, 191, 194

M
Maccoby, Eleanor, 34
Maraboli, Steve, 25
Martin, John, 34
Maturity level, 37
Meals to Remember Template, 204
Meal Theme Nights Template, 205
Medications, weight loss, 83–84
Mental health and eating behavior, 161*t*, 184–187
health concerns and weight and, 186–187
Metabolically healthy obesity, 27–28

Index

Mindful eating, 128
Modeling, 58, 75–76, 82, 105
   and changes involving the entire family, 77–78
Morbidity, 19
Mortality, 19
Musculoskeletal conditions, 144

N

Nature scavenger hunts, 144
Nelson, Jane, 65
Neurodivergent children, 171
Night eating, 161*t*
"No, thank you" bites, 171

O

Obesity
   health problems related to, 12
   metabolically healthy, 27–28
   picky eating and, 162, 169–171
   use of words *obese* and, 27, 64–66
   See also Weight
Outdoor activities, budget-friendly, 144–145

P

Parental eating needs, 161*t*, 181–184
Parenting
   around a child's habits, 36–38
   authoritative, 136
   changes involving the entire family and, 77–78
   changing the family structure for the better, 85–86
   and concerns about children's health and weight, 2–7
   control, strictness, demandingness in, 34–35, 44
   influence on child's development, 33
   modeling and, 75–76, 82, 105
   power struggles in, 164–165
   P & R Coin in, 33, 39–41
   for raising happy and healthy children, 1–2
   scientific approach to, 34–42
   Structure and Love approach to, 42–43
   warmth, acceptance, support in, 34–35
   See also Families
Parks and playgrounds, access to, 16
Personality qualities, focus on positive, 25
Physical activity, 136, 197
   by adolescents, 156
   allergies, asthma, musculoskeletal conditions, or other health conditions preventing, 144

balancing school and homework to include more, 156–157
benefits of, 11
building a schedule for, 154–155
busy family schedules and, 137–138
challenges with electronic use and social media and, 138–140
children and adults enjoying different types of, 147–148
common challenges to, 137–148
family activity ideas for, 141f, 142f, 208–209
health symptoms in caregivers preventing their participation in, 147
increased pressure to engage in more, 146–147
letting children decide how much (or how little) to engage in, 155
limited opportunities near home/limited transportation or money preventing, 144–146
lower interest for child and family in, 140–142
pain or discomfort with, 142–143
for replacing electronics time, 151–152
Structure and Love approach applied to, 46–47
survey on, 201–203
ways to increase family, 153–158
Physical therapists, 144
Pica, 174
Picky eating, 162–163
age of development of, 164
attention-deficit/hyperactivity disorder (ADHD) and, 161t, 176–178
autism spectrum and, 161t, 171–175, 173f
continuing providing one meal for everyone to eat and, 166–167
continuing to eat together for meals and, 166
continuing to offer meals and snacks on schedule and, 165
development of food preferences and, 163
excess weight gain and, 162, 169–171
inviting child to be involved in the process and, 168
learning to trust child and, 168–169
medical conditions to consider with, 161t, 178–180
parental eating needs to consider with, 161t, 181–184
as sensory experience, 175
timed snacks and, 165–166

Planning, meal, 108–111, 193, 204
- at-home meal playbook for, 111–123
- cooking one meal for all and, 121–123
- creating a meal plan for upcoming week in, 113–115
- following through with, 116
- grocery lists for, 116
- planning a day and time for grocery shopping and, 116
- providing foods family enjoys, 123
- sample weekly, 118
- tips for better, 117–118
- when you don't like to cook, 119–120
- writing down list of meals to remember in, 112–113

Play. *See* Physical activity

Positive Discipline: The Classic Guide to Helping Children Develop Self-Discipline, Responsibility, Cooperation, and Problem-Solving Skills, 65

Positive reinforcement, 25–29
Power struggles, 164–165
P & R Coin, 33, 39–41, 98, 193–194
Project EAT, 21

R
Recreation centers, 146
Recreation therapists, 144
Repeated exposure, 57–58
Rudd Center for Food Policy, 64

S
Satter, Ellyn, 40
Satter Eating Competence Model, 40
Satter Feeding Dynamics Model, 40
Schedules
- eating, 104–108, 165, 193, 207
- physical activity, 154–155

Second-order change, 92
Separation, blended families parenting around food during, 95
Shaping, behavior, 152
Simon Says, 145
Sleep, 45, 46*f*, 211
Snacks, 106–107, 125–126
- timed, 165–166

Social media, 138–140
Sole-Smith, Virginia, 63
Structure and Love approach, 42–43, 191, 192–198
- applied to activity, 46–47
- applied to sleep, 45, 46*f*
- family meals and, 47–51

Sustainable health behaviors, 190

T

Teams, families as, 94–96, 100–101
Teasing and bullying, 67–72
Theme nights, planning meal, 115
Times, regular eating, 105–107, 165–166

V

Variety, meal, 110–111
Vegan diets, 161*t*
Vegetarian diets, 161*t*
Veiled health talk, 63
Video games, 145
Visceral fat, 12

W

Walking or running paths, 145
Walking safety, 16
Weekly meal plans, 113–115
Weight
    affirmation of children's bodies and, 23–25
    avoiding talking about, 61–62
    body mass index and, 13–14
    body tendency to stay at same, 17–18, 61
    decision to pursue management of child's, 186–187
    effects of extra, 11–12
    factors affecting, 10–11
    genetics and, 16
    iceberg model of, 14, 15*f*
    impact of words around, 64–66
    influence of environment on, 16–17
    longer-term approach to, 28–29
    overfocus on, 11, 28–29
    positive reinforcement and, 25–29
    use of word, 27
    See also Obesity
Weight loss meal replacements, 161*t*
Weight loss medications, 83–84, 161*t*, 182–183
Wilson, Bee, 163
World Health Organization, 14